Take Control of Your Menopause with a Smart Approach

Dr Ruth Chambers OBE

Professor June Keeling

Professor Fidelma O'Mahony

Dr Bala Sankarasubbu

Rachel Hatfield

Gabby Johnson

Copyright

Cartoons by John Byrne.

ISBN 979-8389154490   Date of publication - April 2023

Disclaimer

Whilst every effort has been made to include accurate and up-to-date information about best practice in managing the menopause and linked digital or healthcare resources such as highlighted websites, knowledge and understanding are constantly evolving and being updated. Therefore, please use the content of this handbook to learn more about how you can adopt or enhance your use of digital healthcare for your own health and wellbeing. Weigh up the choices, information and guidance for your own circumstances. The content is not a substitute for clinical advice from the NHS doctors and nurses who look after you, nor for national advice and guidance given here from professional organisations. Inclusion of named agencies, websites, apps, private companies, services, or publications in this handbook does not constitute a recommendation or endorsement by the co-authors.

Please visit our website https://www.raparu.co.uk/menopause if you want to know more about digital modes of delivery of healthcare and wellbeing that are described in this book.

Acknowledgements

The co-authors are very grateful to Fr John and Paula Stather who've worked really hard to design the book cover and layout, and slot in the cartoons and digital links, so as you'll see, the content is an engaging read.

Contents

Authors   1

Foreword   Rt Hon Caroline Nokes MP   4

Chapter 1   What is this handbook about?   5

Chapter 2   What is the menopause?   11

Chapter 3   Different digital approaches   18

Chapter 4   Improving your lifestyle during
                the menopause   34

Chapter 5   Clinical management of the menopause   64

Chapter 6   Complementary and alternative
                treatments for the menopause   74

Chapter 7   Top tips   83

Chapter 8   Frequently Asked Questions (FAQs)   90

Chapter 9   Make your realistic plan to
                manage your menopause   95

Appendix   QR code links to apps throughout book   102

Authors

Each of the six authors led on writing one or two of the chapters or a lead theme throughout the book, such as digital aids that combat the range of negative effects of the menopause. But we have not attributed particular names to each chapter as much of the contributed material that the co-authors wrote was scattered between chapters too. The first four authors listed below are practising clinicians from a range of health professions providing an inter-disciplinary focus for all the clinical material throughout the book.

Professor Ruth Chambers OBE

Dr Ruth is an honorary professor at Staffordshire University and also Keele University. Dr Ruth recently retired as a practising GP and is on the national temporary emergency medical register still. She has led on digital primary care transformation and quality improvement across Staffordshire general practices; and digital upskilling of clinicians and social workers - creating 800 or so digital champions across England. Ruth has written 81 books (yes 81!!) - mainly for health care teams, some for the public; presented at local events/ national & international conferences; as well as carrying out research, and contributing to national guidance on clinical conditions like cardiovascular disease and lifestyle habits.

Professor June Keeling

June is Professor of Women's Health at Keele University. She lives in the UK and is a Registered General Nurse and Midwife. She has a BSc (Hons) in Women's Health and Health Research from the University of Liverpool, a Masters degree in Professional Education, and a PhD. Her professional background encompasses over forty years of clinical experience, research and writing books. She leads the Women's Health Research group in the School of Nursing and Midwifery, Keele University. Her academic work focuses on the area of women's health including the menopause.

Professor Fidelma O'Mahony

Professor Fidelma graduated from University College Cork (Ireland) and trained as a GP before specialising in Obstetrics & Gynaecology. She was appointed as a Consultant in Obstetrics & Gynaecology and Senior Lecturer in Medical Education in 2003, at the then University Hospitals of North Staffordshire and Keele Medical School. Her clinical interests cover Urogynaecology, Perineal trauma, Paediatric & Adolescent Gynaecology and the Menopause. She supports menopause in the workplace through tri-monthly menopause cafés. She was appointed as Hospital Dean for Keele Medical School at the University Hospitals of North Midlands in 2019 and oversees delivery of undergraduate, medical, physician associate and paramedic education at the Hospital Trust.

Dr Bala Sankarasubbu

Dr Bala is an experienced GP in Staffordshire with specialist interests in Women's Health & Emergency Medicine. She completed postgraduate training in Women's Health, Sexual and Reproductive health, which has allowed her to set up a community women's health clinic in her general practice setting. This has gained lots of positive feedback from her local population. She has also worked as a GP with Special Interest in the A&E department, at Royal Stoke Hospital. She is a GP trainer too, actively involved in postgraduate general practice training. Oh – and Bala enjoys cooking Indian dishes and travelling round the world too!

Rachel Hatfield

Rachel is an experienced digital programme and project manager and has spent the last ten years working in/for the NHS both locally in Staffordshire and Cheshire, and nationally. Rachel currently works for Howbeck Healthcare driving digital upskilling and digital initiatives across the area. Rachel successfully led the national NHS clinician and social care digital upskilling action learning set programme, creating digital clinical champions by developing confidence, capability and capacity for their delivery of accessible technology, empowering NHS staff and patients to improve healthcare outcomes. Rachel has co-authored a number of publications and books related to this work. Previously Rachel spent 10+ years working in the private/retail sector across the UK and Ireland, successfully leading large teams and driving sales.

Gabby Johnson

Gabby is a medical student at the University of Nottingham.
Gabby recently graduated with a Bachelors in Medical Sciences and is continuing her final years of study in Medicine. She has been a part of many projects involving digital technology and how they can improve health across Staffordshire. Gabby has a keen interest in women's health and gynaecology and hopes to pursue this area of medicine in her future career. She recently co-authored the book *Stoke Your Success* - a book that captures the life stories of the many successful people associated with Stoke-on-Trent and nearby locations.

Going Forward:

This book is full of clinical insights and encouragement for any woman to understand and minimise the effects of their menopause, whatever their personal circumstances, at different times in their lives. That might be about improving your lifestyle habits in sustained ways, realising the benefits of hormone replacement therapies or alternative treatments, adopting digital aids so that you have a smart approach to beating your menopause. So complete the action plans in the book, using our hot tips and doctors' insights – in your homelife and at work – as the Rt Hon Caroline Nokes MP describes on the next page.

Foreword

We must tackle the impact on women in the workplace, from the menopause

Over the course of the Women and Equalities Select Committee inquiry into the menopause and the workplace we took evidence from a wide range of employers, legal experts, Trade Unions and women impacted by the menopause.

Their evidence will stay with me forever. Too many women are being forced out of work because of their symptoms, and they are not getting the help they need. It is too difficult to bring a case to tribunal, and frequently they are having to use disability discrimination legislation.

Too many women are being misdiagnosed and prescribed anti-depressants.

Stigma is still prevalent in the workplace, and women are afraid to speak out and ask for help.

That is why the Committee will not let up on this. We need better training for doctors, we need more understanding from employers, and we need legislation that works for menopausal women.

There is hope – the stigma is reducing, we are all being braver about speaking out, more and more employers are introducing workplace menopause policies, and the pre-payment certificate for HRT is being rolled out, making medication much, much cheaper. But there is still work to be done, and I pay credit to all those working and campaigning for how far we have come, and not giving up the fight.

Rt Hon Caroline Nokes MP

Member of Parliament for Romsey and Southampton North
Chair of the UK's Women and Equalities Select Committee

Chapter 1 What is this handbook about?

We hope that this practical handbook will help you to understand and manage your menopause and really get going with using various digital aids to support your self-care to reduce the impact of menopausal symptoms on your health, work and relationships with others. It is thought that around three out of four menopausal women experience related symptoms that affect their personal lives. These symptoms can affect a person's work performance and job satisfaction, as well as their relationships with others, their partner and family members. See Table 9.1 in Chapter 9 for a capture of the very many symptoms and conditions that can be linked to the menopause – you can start ticking off the ones that you think relate to you and those that you're currently experiencing. For instance, hot flushes can go on for decades – but usually do stop within a few years of your last period. But symptoms like a dry vagina or urinary symptoms are likely to persist.

We've tended to focus in this handbook on easily available, accessible and affordable digital aids like apps, and modes of delivery of patient care that are recommended by trustworthy organisations like the NHS or national charities. Not all of the digital aids included here are freely available via NHS or social care providers; but if not, they are reasonably priced and easily bought online or in retail shops or pharmacies. The digital aids we've included throughout this handbook are just examples that we'd recommend to you - but there are lots more apps, devices and online resources available than we have capacity to cover here. So, these are just tasters and you can do more online searching for other alternatives.

What are menopausal symptoms in this period of your life?

Menopause is a natural stage in a woman's life when there is a reduction in her circulating hormone levels. It usually happens between the ages of 45 to 55 years. As women go through their forties (usually) their hormone levels fluctuate – sometimes wildly. And the symptoms of the menopause can be present for many years – before and after someone's periods stop.

Sometimes the menopause can be triggered by other causes such as surgery to remove sexual organs, or chemotherapy treatment for cancer, or a genetic condition.

So, the menopause occurs at the end of your final menstrual period. You'd be described as 'postmenopausal' one year after your last period – as periods have a habit of suddenly re-starting just as you thought you'd seen the last one. But you can suffer from menopausal symptoms over several years whilst you are entering and going through the menopausal phase of your life, as your hormone levels gradually and sporadically dwindle. Most common symptoms include: hot flushes, difficulty sleeping, mood changes, loss of energy, low sex drive (sometimes termed 'loss of libido'), a dry vagina – which can lead to pain or discomfort during sex, and urinary symptoms like stress incontinence.

The usual age for the onset of the menopause – when women start experiencing symptoms - is around 45 to 47 years old onwards; and the average age for having a last period is around 51 years old. It's likely that the age you go through your menopause is similar to what your mother's was.

For many women, menopausal symptoms are mild and can be tolerated without any prescribed treatment. But the numbers of prescriptions given for hormone replacement therapy (HRT) is consistently rising year or year. For instance, in England there was a 35% rise in prescriptions of HRT in 2021/22 (that's 7.8 million prescriptions for 1.93 million identified patients) compared with 2020/21 (when there were 5.9 million prescriptions for 1.48 million patients), according to a recent report from the NHS Business Services Authority.

The most deprived areas had the fewest patients who received an HRT prescription, with almost twice as many patients receiving HRT prescriptions in the least deprived areas of the country – another example of the sad state of health inequalities in the UK. Overall, prescribing of HRT medication was most common for patients aged 50 to 54 years old.

Digital aids that might help you be 'appy

There are a wide range of digital aids that can help you to understand more about your symptoms of the menopause and guide you towards ways to minimise the effects of your menopause and allied health issues and/or improving your lifestyle habits. These will include trustworthy apps, video-consultation with a clinician, social media channel such as WhatsApp or Facebook, telehealth or texting, online learning resources on recommended websites, digital access to your own medical records held by your general practice, or your ability to book clinical appointments online.

People are increasingly choosing to book appointments at their general practice and order repeat prescriptions online. Some want to view their own health records online, including blood test results and medical histories, and speak to their doctor or nurse by a video link, via apps on their smartphones or tablets. This should enable individuals to make informed decisions about their health and wellbeing. But there are potential risks too – for example some people found their GP or nurse to be too remote and inaccessible during the COVID-19 pandemic.

People might be coerced by family members or friends to share access to their medical records with potential harm and safeguarding issues if there is sensitive information in the content (for instance, notes relating to a previous termination of pregnancy that the patient had not disclosed to others). If online services are the prime way to book a consultation at a GP practice, those who are more technologically able might snap up the majority of appointments at the expense of people who live without home internet access, or are not digitally competent. There is a problem too that in some homes, couples may use the same email address if one or both are technology-challenged with their skills or enthusiasm to use digital communication; so that means their privacy might be breached by their partner who might be able to view their email correspondence and access their medical records.

Nowadays in GP practices and other NHS settings, digital consultation should be offered as a standard service unless there are good clinical reasons (or patient preferences) to select other modes of consultation. Here are some ways that are likely to be available to you to find out more about the treatment you are offered, or provided with, for your menopause:

- online consultations that can be used by patients (or their carers on their behalf) to enable their general practice team to allocate patients accessing the online consultation platform, the right service (in person, phone, email, video-call or simply a prescription or advice) for their health problem(s) (e.g. sending in their current blood pressure readings for a nurse to review and send an online response back) and personal needs.
- a video-consultation between patient (or their carer) and clinician; or even a regular video-group meeting organised by a practice nurse for several women suffering from menopausal symptoms to share experiences and tips.
- two-way secure written communication emailed between patient (or their carer) and practice.
- an up-to-date accessible online presence, such as a website, that links to an online consultation system and other online services.
- signposting to a validated symptom checker and self-care health information (e.g. nhs.uk).
- shared record access between clinicians and a patient, including patients being able to add text to the content of their medical record, as well as being able to read it online.
- online access for a patient (or their carer) to request prescriptions such as their HRT medication.
- online appointment booking with a practice nurse and/or GP.
- an online method to inform their practice of a change of address, contact details, or other demographic information.

A remote consultation may be less appropriate than a face-to-face one if you are severely ill, have a mix of health conditions that impact on each other, are visually impaired, have poor English language skills (and access to an online interpreter is difficult), have learning disabilities or autism, or difficulties operating technology, like a smartphone.

Successful consulting depends on both the clinician and you as a patient having access to a private space and a reliable digital setup.

As you start to read this handbook why not capture how ready you feel you are to use the technology such as the smartphone you already have and use in your personal life…for your health and wellbeing? Then after you've read through the rest of the handbook and engaged in looking at the information and resources in the next chapters relevant to the menopause and any other health condition(s) – take the survey again. Hopefully it won't take much effort to realise that there are many digital opportunities that are easily accessed and already available to you – to improve your lifestyle habits, cope better with the menopause, or boost your health and personal wellbeing. So, answer the four questions in Table 1.1 below, and keep a record of your answers – thinking how can you improve your scores?

Table 1.1 Digital literacy survey for you to take – how smart are you?			
1. How often do you use digital technology e.g. apps, texting - in your personal life or at work?	25% or less	About 50% of the time	75% or more	Never
2. Which of the following statements most closely describes how you feel in relation to using digital technology for say video-consultation?	'Digitally Worried' I can see the benefits of new ways but they often make me nervous.	'Digitally Ready' I feel comfortable with the digital world and have the skills to adapt to the changes.	'Digitally Leading' I love adapting to change and embrace digital opportunities for aiding my health & wellbeing.
3. To what extent do you agree with the following statement? 'I can see the benefit of using digital aids for my health care and wellbeing'	Disagree	Neutral	Somewhat agree	Strongly agree
4. To what extent do you agree with the following statement? 'I can see the benefit of using digital aids for my menopause and reducing the effects on me'	Disagree	Neutral	Neutral	Strongly agree

And what about your confidence and competence to use a range of digital aids that you have access to? Take the test and add your answers to Table 1.2 too:

Table 1.2 Digital competency survey for you to take			I feel confident	I feel a little confident	I don't feel at all confident
Competence	When I want to:	Search the internet			
		Use apps			
		Download an app			
Can-do Attitude	When on an app, if things don't go right first time, I am prepared to keep at it to sort it out...				
Communication	When I want to contact family and friends by:	Texts			
		Phone calls			
		Facetime/video calls			
Comprehension	When I need to use apps, I can usually find my way around:				
Capability	When I get a new device and have to set it up by myself:	Phone			
		Laptop			
		Tablet			

Actions! So, if you've not scored 'high marks' in Table 1.1 and/or Table 1.2, what's your plan to improve your digital literacy and competency to be able to optimise your use of digital aids to understand more about your menopause, or find ways to help you overcome its effects?

Chapter 2 What is the menopause?

The menopause is the time in a woman's life when she stops having periods. It occurs when the ovaries stop producing the hormones: oestrogen, progesterone and testosterone. For most women this happens between the ages of 45 -55 years, and symptoms can last for several years. The term 'menopause transition' is frequently used to describe all stages of the menopause. There are a range of different symptoms that women might experience during their menopause transition. As well as changes to the pattern of their periods, most women experience a range of other associated symptoms such as hot flushes, anxiety and mood swings (tick off yours on the list given in Table 9.1 in Chapter 9). These symptoms can last for months or years; and can change with time. Maybe a person gets hot flushes and night sweats and they start to improve, but a low mood and anxiety might then feature more as the months or years, go by.

In some cases, menopausal symptoms begin when a woman's periods stop suddenly. For other women it is not quite so obvious, and they might experience symptoms of the menopause while still having periods. Or it may be that changes in the pattern of their periods are the very first symptom of the menopause that a woman experiences. Bleeding may get lighter or heavier, and happen less often or more often.

Developing symptoms of the menopause while still having periods is called the 'perimenopause'. The **perimenopause** includes the time beginning with the first features of the approaching menopause, such as hot flushes or menstrual irregularity, which can appear years before a woman's periods actually stop. It ends 12 months after the last menstrual period. The **postmenopause** starts with the last menstrual period but cannot be dated with certainty until 12 months have gone by without any periods recurring.

A **premature menopause** is usually defined as the permanent cessation of menstrual periods due to loss of ovarian follicular activity occurring before a woman reaches 40 years of age; it is officially termed '**premature ovarian insufficiency**' or POI.

POI can happen for a medical reason - after surgery, where a woman's ovaries have been removed, or following cancer treatments such as radiotherapy or chemotherapy. It can sometimes be associated with other health conditions, such as severe eating disorders. However, in many cases there is no medical reason. POI can affect not just someone's periods but also their fertility, heart disease or bone health, and so input from a relevant specialist may be required.

An **early menopause** is when the ovaries stop functioning between 40-45 years old, in the absence of any other secondary causes of periods stopping, such as chemotherapy. Around one in 100 women in the UK experience an early menopause.

A **surgical menopause** occurs when the ovaries are removed; this is sometimes done alongside a hysterectomy and causes a sudden drop in female hormone levels, often triggering severe symptoms.

There is no need for blood tests to diagnose the menopause in women after the age of 45 years old. The diagnosis can be made from the nature of their symptoms. However, it may be necessary in some cases to exclude other medical problems if the picture is not clear. So, the blood test serum follicle-stimulating hormone (FSH) should not be used to diagnose the perimenopause or menopause in healthy women aged over 45 years old with typical symptoms of the menopause. But it may be used to test a woman under 40 years old with suspected premenstrual ovarian insufficiency, or if a woman is aged 40-45 years old with menopausal symptoms, or aged over 45 years with atypical symptoms.

For women under the age of 45 years, and particularly for those under 40 years of age, blood tests are useful. Hormone levels should be re-checked six weeks apart to help to reach a reliable diagnosis.

Overall, now that we are all living longer most women will live more than a third of their life after their menopause. Because menopausal symptoms can have a significant impact on women's health and well being, there has been an increasing interest in taking hormone replacement therapy (HRT) (read more about this in Chapter 5).

Symptoms of the menopause - it's a long list

Menopausal symptoms vary widely from woman to woman, as does the length of time they last. Around 75% of women will experience menopause symptoms and on average these last up to seven years. However, studies suggest that up to one third of women experience symptoms for longer than this, and for some that can be into their 60s and beyond.

Symptoms can be classified as follows:

- Vasomotor symptoms: these are hot flushes and night-time sweats. About 70-80% of women experience these symptoms. This in turn can lead to insomnia, exhaustion and anxiety.
- Cognitive symptoms and mood disorders: these describe the mental health and psychological symptoms associated with the menopause. They include brain fog, poor concentration, memory loss, irritability, lack of confidence, low mood and anxiety. If women already have mental health problems such as depression and anxiety, these can be made worse at the time of their menopause.
- Musculoskeletal problems: these include muscle and joint aching and pain. It often occurs in the morning and can affect the woman's existing joint problems. It leads to tiredness and can interfere with day to day activities such as taking exercise and work activities.
- Fatigue, tiredness and low energy: these may be a specific feature of the menopause but may also be the result of poor sleep due to other symptoms.
- Sleep disturbance and insomnia: as we age our sleep pattern changes. However due to hormonal changes this can be worse during the menopause, despite good sleep hygiene. In addition, sleep disturbance may be made worse due to night-time sweats or mood disorders. Then such disturbed sleep may trigger fatigue, irritability or loss of concentration in the day.
- Loss of, or reduced, sexual desire and libido: women's testosterone levels begin to decrease gradually over time, starting before the time of their menopause. While low testosterone levels can cause a loss of libido there may be other causes too,

including relationship difficulties, vaginal dryness, and general menopausal symptoms which may also be causal factors.

- Genitourinary symptoms: these include vaginal dryness and burning or irritation and can result in pain on intercourse. In addition, there may be cystitis (inflammation of the bladder often caused by a urinary infection) with increased frequency and pain on passing urine. Some women experience recurrent lower urinary tract infections (UTIs). These symptoms often present later in life, and can be many years after the menopause after other symptoms have settled.

- Reduced quality of life: menopausal symptoms can have a negative impact on people's overall wellbeing and impact on their quality of life. Women may have difficulties in coping with the demands of a job they have previously managed successfully. Unsurprisingly relationships very often suffer due to the distressing nature of menopausal symptoms. In addition, menopause symptoms can lead to a woman's loss of enjoyment of life and maybe stop them from participating in their usual hobbies, and social or family events.

Health risks – but it's not a life sentence!

The menopause can have an impact on a woman's long-term health too. Some conditions are directly linked with a fall in oestrogen levels, such as developing osteoporosis and heart disease. In addition, pre-existing health conditions often get worse at this time.

Osteoporosis occurs when a person's bones become more fragile and less dense. This begins at the time of the menopause because the bones of the female skeleton rely on oestrogen for their strength. Bone is made of an outer shell (or cortex) which becomes thin; and an inner mesh (trabeculae), which loses its strength. For some women a fracture or broken bone, may be the first sign that they have of osteoporosis. These fractures may cause pain and disability. In particular, this can affect the bones in the spine (vertebrae) leading to loss of height and changes in shape, such as 'dowager's hump' which results in a bent-over position.

The risk of developing osteoporosis increases as we get older. There are a number of health, dietary and lifestyle factors which affect the increased risk of osteoporosis. Women who have an early menopause (or POI) are at greater risk. Women with some underlying medical conditions such as inflammatory bowel disorders, (ulcerative colitis or Crohn's disease), coeliac disease or some forms of arthritis, will have a greater risk of osteoporosis. An increased risk of osteoporosis is also associated with some drugs, which are essential treatments for other medical conditions. These include long-term steroid tablets and some cancer treatments.

Osteoporosis is also more likely to occur as a result of adverse lifestyle habits such as smoking, drinking more than 10-14 units of alcohol per week, binge drinking, and lack of exercise.

Diet plays an important part in sustaining bone health. Calcium and vitamin D are both essential for bones and so having a poor diet lacking in calcium and vitamin D will increase a person's likelihood of developing osteoporosis.

As we get older, we have an increased risk of developing cardiovascular or heart disease. This increased risk coincides with the onset of the menopause, due to a lack of oestrogen. There is also a tendency to put on weight and to develop diabetes in middle age. If a person already has a family history of heart disease and diabetes these risks are increased further. Again, adverse lifestyle factors such as a poor diet, lack of exercise, obesity, smoking and alcohol consumption can increase those risks.

At the time of the menopause there are numerous other health issues and symptoms which women encounter. So, while menopause is clearly a factor, a lack of oestrogen is not the only thing that causes health conditions like heart disease or diabetes. And so, an overall review of their health and lifestyle is needed to manage or treat women well, in their mid-life or older lifetime.

Doctors' insights:

Gill (43 years old) came to see her GP as she thought she was going through the 'change'. She was still having regular periods – sometimes they were heavy and at other times short. She was feeling tired and sometimes got hot flushes. She had been sterilised several years previously, and her blood pressure and weight were in the ideal ranges. She wasn't able to confirm when her mum had gone through the change. Her GP carried out some blood tests which her normal hormone levels showed that she wasn't going through the menopause. But other blood tests showed that her iron and folic acid levels were both too low – which meant that Gill needed to take replacements. Her GP arranged an ultrasound scan of her abdomen too to investigate the cause of her heavy periods (the scan turned out to be normal).

Doctor's insights: consider getting blood tests done through your general practice to see if you need to take multivitamins, if you think you're starting to suffer from the menopause but are still having regular periods. Your GP will consider if they need to arrange a scan of your abdomen to check if there might be another cause of your menstrual symptoms.

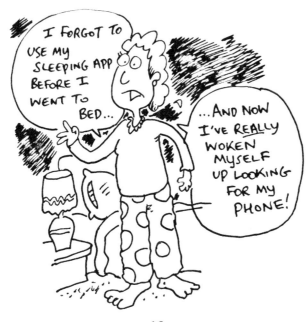

Jackie (43 years old) had irregular and heavy periods, and arranged to consult her GP because of the brain fog she was suffering, that she thought was affecting her daily activities. Her mum, aunt and grandma had each experienced the menopause in their early 40s. She was complaining of tiredness, being forgetful and was snappy at home with her family. But she denied having any undue stress at home or work. Her children were aged 14 and 11 years old. Her hormonal blood test for the menopause (FSH) was normal. Her last period was three months ago. Her abdominal scan, blood pressure and body mass index (BMI) were all normal. Her GP came to a provisional diagnosis of suspected early menopause and sought advice from a specialist gynaecology clinic. The specialist advised her to start on a combined HRT patch and was keen for her to be seen for follow-up in the menopause clinic.

Doctor's insights: as Jackie is aged 43 years old, she is at the 'early menopause' stage. She could consider taking vitamin D daily which she can buy over the counter - as premature or early menopause can cause thinning of the bones (termed 'osteoporosis') and regular vitamin D supplementation can help to prevent this.

Chapter 3 Different digital approaches

There are many trusted apps, sources of online information from reliable websites, wearable tech, digital modes like video calls that can help someone to learn more about the menopause, or help them to deal with the effects, or prevent worsening of their health conditions. So, the content of this chapter should help you to engage, by highlighting personal gains that you might get from using such digital aids. Please read through the disclaimer at the start of the book as a reminder that inclusion of named agencies, websites, apps, private companies, services, or publications in this handbook does not constitute a recommendation or endorsement of the resource by the authors.

Many women going through the menopause can suffer from psychosocial symptoms. These symptoms can increase the risks of them developing anxiety and/or depression, as well as causing body and self-identity issues as a result of the physical changes experienced during this time. This can lead to a loss of confidence, or increased stress levels affecting all aspects of their life – such as their performance at work and behaviour at home. These feelings can affect their physical and mental health and impact on all aspects of their life. Using digital technology can empower women to get the information and support that they need, when they need it, in a way that suits them. Everyone's journey is unique to them as an individual and the approach to manage the diverse effects from their menopause needs to reflect that.

Digital technologies provide different ways to access information and support in 'safe' ways; for example, someone may want to engage with their peers and others going through the same experience, whilst being able to remain anonymous. Or, they may want to speak to their health professional but struggle to attend a face to face appointment due to personal time constraints from their working patterns, or family commitments. Some women may want to look at alternative ways to control/manage their menopausal symptoms but find the volume of conflicting information overwhelming and need some guidance on where to start.

Digital technologies can support women in different ways, and individuals can use what is relevant and useful to them. The menopause and how it affects individuals varies by person so there is no one size fits all approach. As discussed elsewhere in the book there are a lot of complicated feelings, adverse reactions and taboos surrounding the menopause and the huge variety of symptoms that many women suffer.

Apps - getting a helping hand

Many people rely on apps on their smartphone/tablet to access information and use that to manage aspects of their health and well-being. An app (short for 'application') is a type of software available on most smartphones, tablets and newer versions of Windows, that combines features (such as information/images) together, to inform and empower the user. They are downloaded directly to a smart device via the operating system's store (e.g. Google Play on Android devices or the App store on Apple devices). There are a multitude of apps available today, with the most commonly downloaded types being health/lifestyle apps, gaming apps, social media apps, news apps, shopping/utility apps and productivity apps.

People tend to use apps as they are easy to access, simple to download and usually available to be used whenever the person wants them. Apps are often customisable to the user so offering a personalised experience. Information can be saved and adapted to the user's requirements. They usually offer both online and offline capabilities, meaning that they are much more accessible for the user and they can be accessed almost anywhere, and at any time. Information is often current and can be updated by the provider a lot quicker than more traditional methods. Once the update is complete the app reflects this. This is great for health apps which may require to be regularly updated with new information being published or a change in national guidance.

With the use of a smartphone or tablet device you can download apps to assist you with the self-care and self-management of your health at home. The NHS (NHS Better Heath) and Public Health England have accredited a number of apps for a variety of health conditions and ORCHA's AppFinder (developed with clinicians) is commissioned by a number of local health organisations and councils in the UK to support people with identifying suitable, useful and trustworthy apps for their health and wellbeing. It independently reviews apps across all health and wellbeing conditions and provides a breakdown of each review matched to its key assessment criteria; which include clinical assurance, data privacy and user experience.

You can read other people's reviews of an app (if available) to provide an overview of content/relevance and user feedback, prior to downloading a particular app.

Some apps are free, some are free with paid features included and some incur a cost to download, so be sure to only download ones with which you feel comfortable.

Balance app/website: The Balance app, created by Dr Louise Newson allows users to track their symptoms in a journal, participate in a community with others, and guides the user to access articles to read more about the menopause, various treatments and advice. The app is personalised to each individual where you can add your various health conditions and circumstances, so that articles shared with you are relevant to you.

The app is free for access to the basic features; but the app will prompt you to set up a free account using your email address and ask for some personal details so that the app can be personalised for you. You can also pay to upgrade to the Balance+ option which gives access to premium features such as learning more about how you can tailor your food, sleep and mood as well access to top experts in the field with live sessions where you can ask questions. This premium version of the app is available as an in-app purchase.

https://www.balance-menopause.com/

Videos that can also be found in the Balance Menopause Library: https://www.balance-menopause.com/menopause-library/

This resource is suitable for: perimenopause, postmenopause, premature and surgical menopause

---

Suzanne (aged 50 years old) tells how the Balance app helped her

"Balance has been my helping hand throughout the menopause and has helped me to keep a track of my symptoms and be able to relay these to my doctor easily. I personally really struggle to cope with my hot flushes, my low mood and vaginal dryness. To combat these I have used the Balance app to review my treatment options such as HRT and how they may help me, read up about hormones and the role they play in my body, and why I am feeling the way that I do. I am now looking to commence HRT with my doctor now that I feel better informed, thanks to my Balance app. I can easily show my doctor my symptom log via the app; that is an accurate representation of me and how I have been feeling. I have recommended the Balance app to my friends and I encourage anyone to give it a go!"

Health & Her app/website: Health & Her is designed to help you to track your symptoms, triggers and changes in your monthly cycle, whilst offering support and recommending some supplements that can be purchased through them 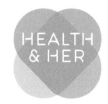 directly. Whilst using *Health & Her* you can set personal goals and learn from top experts in the field by reading their articles and advice.

The app is free, but the app will prompt you to create a free account using your email address and ask for some personal details, so that the app will be personalised. All the content is free to use but the products advertised are not - such as supplements which can be purchased directly from *Health & Her*.

https://healthandher.com/

This resource is suitable for: perimenopause, postmenopause and surgical menopause.

Caria app: Caria allows users to explore how to manage symptoms and treatment options, to get involved in community discussions, set daily goals to improve your health whilst logging symptoms and triggers and listening to a range of audios as to how you might get instant relief from your menopausal symptoms.

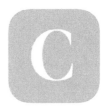

The Caria app gives you a breakdown of all medications, supplements and alternative therapies used for the menopause to enable you to make an informed decision of what may work well for you that you might want to try.

The app is free for the basic features but will prompt you to set up a free account using your email address and ask for some personal details so that the app can be personalised. You can upgrade to Caria Premium which gives you access to premium features such as unlimited access to additional content such as recipes, guides and online classes. This is an in-app purchase. This app is only available on the Apple Appstore at the current time, and not on Google Play.

Vicky (aged 56 years old) tells her story of how the Caria app helped her

"When I first became menopausal I was not sure where to look for information or advice to guide me on my menopausal journey. I came across many apps; my personal favourite is Caria. Caria is so broad in the range of options that it offers. I like to use the nightly stretch routines each evening to relax but they also help to manage my symptoms. Symptom relief is something that I found very difficult at the start but the guides on Caria for instant help get me through the tough patches when I need to. When I wanted to learn more I read one of the articles which explained what the menopause was and what to expect. I had no idea of what was normal and what was not beforehand, and this has helped me to better understand my body. Caria has helped me to take control of my body and my experiences of my menopausal symptoms."

Perry app/website: the Perry app allows users to connect with other like minded women in the 'Sisters' Chat' to share advice and ask questions, look at resources such as articles and podcasts and promotes a safe environment. Perry also promotes products to combat a variety of menopausal related symptoms, such as skin changes but these come at an additional charge.

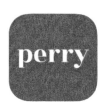

The app is free, but the app will prompt you to set up a free account using your email address and ask for some personal details so that the app can be personalised. All the content is free to use but the products advertised are not - such as supplements which can be purchased directly (please note that the costings of these products are advertised in US dollars).

This information is also available on the website: https://heyperry.com

This is suitable for: perimenopause

MenoLife app: The MenoLife app allows users to track their health and wellbeing in relation to their menstrual cycles, sleep and exercise. There are articles to explore other topics such as food, beauty and symptom relief along with videos from experts in the field. MenoLife offers mindfulness tools too, to provide relief and relaxation.

The app is free, but the app will prompt you to set up a free account using your email address and telephone number and ask for some personal details so that the app can be personalised. All the content is free to use but the products advertised are not - such as supplements which would be purchased directly (please note that the costings of these products are advertised in US dollars).

This is suitable for: perimenopause and postmenopause

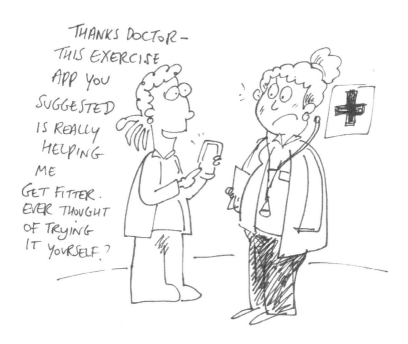

Trustworthy websites – the right path

You might go to national/well known websites to learn more about health and wellbeing or lifestyle choices. There are millions of websites dedicated to specific conditions and search engines will identify relevant websites in a matter of seconds.

Just like apps, websites are a great way to access the information and support when you need it. The information is available instantly online and in a variety of accessible formats. So, you don't need to make an appointment or schedule time to speak to someone as everything can be accessed in your own time, when you need it. As with all internet-based information though make sure that you check the information you are accessing or referring to is from a trusted site or source.

The Menopause Charity website: The Menopause Charity website is founded by Dr Louise Newson and looks at various aspects of the menopause, such as hormone replacement therapy (HRT), symptoms, living well with the menopause and many more topics - in the form of articles on the website. There are also articles with tailored expert advice on many subjects such as the advantages of yoga, or healthy eating.

The website content is free to access with no sign up needed unless you want to be kept informed about the Charity's progress and news. There is also the opportunity to donate to the Charity. Healthcare workers can access training through the Charity too, if they are interested in learning more.

www.themenopausecharity.org

It is suitable for: perimenopause and postmenopause

Menopause and Me website: The Menopause and Me website provides information on all types of treatment available for the menopause, the changes that may happen to the woman's body and the stages of the menopause. There are a variety of options to find information such as via podcasts, or access to a glossary of terms and an interactive symptoms checklist. These resources are designed to help you when discussing your menopausal journey with a healthcare professional.

The Menopause and Me site is unique in that it provides links to other sources of information such as for younger women and their menopause, and the International Menopause society.

The website content is free to access with no sign up needed. The website also allows you to request a free copy of their guidebooks to gain more information.

https://www.menopauseandme.co.uk/

It is suitable for: perimenopause, postmenopause and premature menopause.

Women's Health Concern website: The Women's Health Concern (WHC) site is the patient accessible part of the British Menopause Society website and provides a confidential and independent service to advise and reassure women about their gynaecological, sexual and post-reproductive health.

The women's health concern area is useful as it has a range of fact sheets that you can access and download, on different aspects concerning the menopause, as well as more on the information included in the content of the videos being discussed by experts.

The website content is free to access with no sign up needed. The website does however signpost health products that may come at a cost if you want to buy them, as well as a link to donate to the Charity.

https://www.womens-health-concern.org/

It is suitable for: perimenopause, postmenopause and premature menopause

Video Consultations - heads up

Video consultations are now being increasingly offered by health professionals alongside traditional face to face or telephone appointment options and are a great way to engage, and discuss your symptoms/concerns about the menopause, with a health professional. So, this is a consultation carried out using your smartphone, tablet or computer. Although video consultations may not be suitable for everyone, they can often be a lot easier for some people to attend, rather than face to face appointments. For example, many working age women may struggle to get time off work to attend routine NHS appointments - the travel and waiting time combined can often be much longer than the consultation itself.

Virtual consultations allow more flexibility. They can be taken at a convenient time wherever the person feels comfortable, with good connectivity and a private area. Often the menopause triggers multiple symptoms and being prepared in advance of meeting with a healthcare professional allows someone to be clear when discussing these. Attending the general practice surgery in person can increase someone's stress; and video consultations often decrease this stress, allowing the consultation to be more focussed.

Make sure that you have a quiet and private space to take the video call. If another person is present in your room, introduce them to your health professional; as they should do if there is another person in their consultation room. You both need to consent to others being present.

You may be asked to confirm your personal details e.g. name and date of birth to ensure that you are the patient for whom they have medical records open. Your health professional will be taking notes as your consultation progresses. They cannot digitally record your conversation without your explicit permission. Similarly, if you want to record your consultation, you should ask the health professional you're connected with if that's okay.

Video Group Consultations - you're in good company

Virtual group consultations deliver routine care to groups of patients online, consulting with patients who have the same or similar health condition and challenges, such as the menopause. This is by delivering an adapted online version of face-to-face group consultations, which still enables the delivery of routine care including clinical, lifestyle advice, prescription changes and reassurance.

People can receive clinical and educational advice and guidance via video group consultations from their clinical facilitator, whilst also getting advice, input and support from other patients in the group - a great way to receive peer support from other women in a similar situation to you. This promotes a better understanding of a person's condition, how others are managing, a space to share experiences and learning with others, going through the same thing in a safe setting.

Everyone participating should realise that they are part of a confidential discussion and should not take screenshots or record the session. This is implied by you accepting the invite and entering the video group menopause session in a trusting way. A recent trial of a virtual group consultation for menopause treatment in London worked out really well. As many as 25 women with menopausal symptoms joined in most of the weekly sessions (18 were from ethnic minority backgrounds and/or lived in a deprived area – so there was a good mix of women taking part), led by GPs. They were given access to further virtual group meetings with a dietitian or woman's health physiotherapist as required. Their menopause-specific quality of life scores improved by over 50% - a great success.

Rebecca (aged 58 years old) tells how well being part of an online video group with other women suffering from their menopause worked for her

"I tried many ways to manage my symptoms and I hated being alone in this journey. I wanted to connect with others who understood my situation, and in whom I could confide. When I found a video group consultation focussing on the menopause which was led by a local nurse who was a real expert on the menopause, I was delighted as this was exactly what I was looking for! I was truly a part of a community and I felt supported by my fellow ladies and this kept my spirits high. As well as having the support of women in a similar situation, I also had the support of my GP, dietitians and many others - so it was the best of all worlds!"

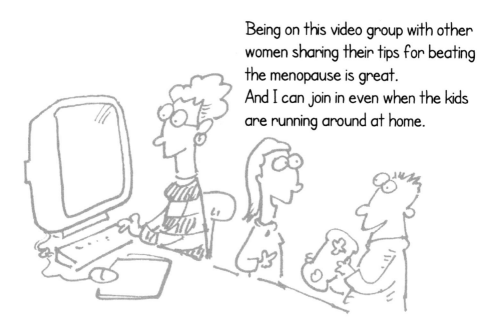

Being on this video group with other women sharing their tips for beating the menopause is great.
And I can join in even when the kids are running around at home.

Health Professional to Patient Texting - put your finger on it

Following interactions with health professionals, many now follow up with their patients using texting systems to share information. This enables them to easily share links to suitable websites, recommend apps or literature about a condition and this interaction is much easier via texts. People can access the information provided as and when they choose - at a time that is convenient to them and beneficial to them as a patient.

Sending information in this format is much more accessible than circulating leaflets by post or face-to-face in a consultation, as more details can be shared that can enable further follow up between clinician and patient, as required. Sharing information that people can access when they need it is much more inclusive than the old style medical practice, when a patient had to fit in with the doctor's or nurse's availability.

Social Media - Face up to the effects of your menopause

Social media platforms provide great ways of sharing/accessing information such as useful guidance, links to apps and websites and general advice. People are able to interact with various platforms to manage their health and wellbeing. Some GP surgeries and hospitals use public Facebook pages to inform people of services that are available, health campaigns, health education and promotion. Apps often have linked social media accounts where people can join to gain additional information and engage with others.

There are regulated and unregulated open and closed Facebook pages and groups dedicated to specific health conditions, providing a forum for people to exchange information and receive peer support - but without them sharing their private and personal details. Using social media is another way of promoting people's independence and self-management. These platforms often create a safe space for individuals to discuss their health/adverse lifestyle issues, whilst remaining as anonymous as they want. Peer support can be a huge benefit to improving people's mental health too.

There are many menopause support groups already out there that women can join which have been created and managed by local and national organisations/ charities/hospitals or individuals experiencing the same thing. A simple search on social media for *menopause* brings up a multitude of closed and public pages/groups that individuals can request to join.

Again, a one size all approach does not fit all; people need to join and try out different groups and see which (if any) are suitable for them and provide the support that they need, want or hope for. Members of these groups can share real life examples and experiences too.

Groups can often encourage new sufferers to look forward and gain positivity, as members offer real peer support and sharing what has worked for them; providing positivity that there are options to manage the menopause that are available that work.

Social media is a great way to find out more about improved lifestyle choices too and make important contacts to get support for many related issues. It can be used for signposting to other lifestyle information and choices that can have a positive impact on a person's quality of life if they take it up and boost their confidence in managing to live through their own menopause.

Animations - get the picture?

Animations are an accessible way of sharing information with people. Many large organisations such as NHS, Public Health England, Councils and the Government use animations to share information and key messages with members of the public. Offering information in different formats makes it more accessible and appealing so that the person putting the messages out there can engage with a wide audience. It can be difficult to absorb all the information around a health condition in a short consultation or from a leaflet. So, animations are a feature that allow people to watch and return to look again, as and when they want to learn more from the messages, and make a plan to adopt some of the advice or copy other people's recommended activities.

Wearable technology - your personal aid

The range and use of wearable technology for self-monitoring of health and wellbeing is vast and evolving constantly. Wearable technology supports the user to understand their body or health condition better, and take more control by empowering them to self-care. Wearable devices often gather usable data through numerous sensors providing insights into a person's activity or other aspects of their health, that is conveyed into a device that they wear on their body, like a sensitive watch.

Knowledge about symptoms and insights into appropriate responses, can be a powerful tool for anyone suffering with a specific condition such as the menopause, or just wanting to increase their wellbeing through a healthy lifestyle. Many wearable aids capture information and identify personal trends, so maybe the person notices that a particular symptom happens at the same time each month – maybe related to the timing of their periods. This knowledge and the associated insights can be very powerful to someone who is suffering a range of symptoms and unsure as to how to manage these intelligently.

Many women going through the menopause find that taking regular exercise supports both their health and wellbeing; and many wearable technology devices feature step counts and related exercise achieved (read more in Chapter 4).

Personal digital assistants

Personal digital assistants such as the Amazon Alexa can support people with their health and wellbeing. Most utilise voice recognition which can be used to support individuals. Some are audio speakers and some have screens so information can be accessed across different formats.
These can be really useful for accessing a range of information when needed - for example accessing online workouts developed for specific health benefits, getting recipe ideas to support good nutrition and healthy eating.

Listening to podcasts of others experiencing the same things in their lives and their positive actions may help someone to realise that they are not the only person suffering like this.

And so.............

Not everyone feels comfortable in discussing how they are feeling or the effects that the menopause is having on them with a health professional, maybe feeling that they won't be taken seriously. So, using digital tools in a non-judgemental way to find out more personal information, reviewing or comparing their symptoms, accessing practical information that they can use to support them to manage their own condition, really helps to manage their health more effectively and efficiently.

So that might be by getting and receiving information from health professionals via video consultations, video group consultations, and text messaging, or accessing independently available apps and websites for their specific and general health/wellbeing information. Making access to information accessible and more available empowers people to manage their menopause and many aspects of their health more effectively and efficiently.

Health/wellbeing apps/websites/community groups provide detailed information in easy-to-understand bitesize pieces, and allow people to refer back to the information as and when they need it, getting support from others experiencing the same or similar issues in real time.

Chapter 4
Improving your lifestyle during the menopause

'Mastering' your Menopause - hot news

If you know yourself, or have been told you are 'menopausal' you may be experiencing a wide range of physical and psychological changes. These can affect your everyday life including family relationships and working ones. You may feel that this is a challenging time as your body functions in a different way to the one you are used to, with loss of menstruation, mood changes and 'brain fog'. Think positively and believe you can 'Master' your menopause. Try and invest in yourself *every* day doing something that makes you feel good about yourself. Mental health and physical health are inter-related, so one will impact on the other. There are several approaches that can support you and ease this transition. Take a look at the diagram below, showcasing how elements of your health and wellbeing overlap and interact.

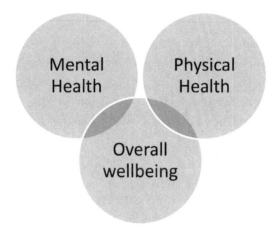

Weight management - waist not, want not

Have you heard the phrase 'middle aged spread?' Well, this often refers to the weight that women gain at that age. Changes in hormone levels might make you more likely to gain weight, but weight gain is also due to eating more calories than your body requires. Other factors include lack of physical activity, unhealthy eating and poor sleep, all of which might contribute to menopausal weight gain.

Obesity is a medical condition diagnosed when someone's BMI (body mass index) is greater than 30kg/m^2. It is important to remember that obesity is a clinical term with specific health implications, and not a judgement on a person's appearance.

A person's body mass index does not distinguish exactly between the relative proportions of their body fat and their muscles. Nor does it take account of the distribution of fat around their body. Some people who might not be defined as obese according to their BMI measure, may still have a high degree of abdominal obesity, also termed 'central' obesity.

A person's BMI is a simple index of weight-for-height that is used to classify how overweight they are, to estimate the proportion of fat in their body (their adiposity) as a rough guide. The same measure is used for both sexes and all ages of adults. People who have a high level of muscle mass (usually young men) may incorrectly be placed in the overweight category, so any BMI measure must be interpreted with caution.

People from an Asian population appear to suffer worse health consequences with the same BMI measure than Caucasians do. So, a BMI of 23kg/m^2 and above is classified as being above the ideal range for someone of South Asian ethnicity living in the UK, as opposed to a BMI of 25kg/m^2 and above for Caucasians – which are the BMI levels classed as being 'overweight'.

The higher risks of developing health conditions such as heart disease, musculoskeletal disorders and some cancers – described as 'co-morbidities' are shown in the Box 4.1 on the following page:

Box 4.1: Classification and risk

Classification and risk of overweight in adults according to their BMI (for the Caucasian population)		
Classification	*BMI (kg/m²)*	*Risk of co-morbidities*
Underweight	< 18.5	Low (but risk of other health problems increased; and may be due to serious illness)
Desirable (ideal) range	18.5–24.9	Average
Overweight	25.0–29.9	Increased
Obesity class I	30.0–34.9	Moderate
Obesity class II	35.0–39.9	Severe
Obesity class III (also known as 'morbid' obesity)	≥ 40.0	Very severe

An adult's waist circumference is an important measure in assessing the extent to which a person is overweight, and their waist:hip ratio too. In fact, the relative distribution of fat between waist and hip predicts someone's likelihood of developing future heart disease or diabetes, better than their body mass index does.

Have a go at measuring your waist:hip ratio. Measure your waist at its narrowest point and your hips at their widest point. Put the tape measure around your waist, firmly, but not digging in, half-way between your lowest rib and the bony top of your pelvis - it will be just above your tummy button (umbilicus). Relax and breathe out naturally, then take the measurement. Repeat the measurement to make sure that you got it right.

In general, target values for adults are less than 0.95 waist/hip ratio for men, and less than 0.85 waist/hip ratio for women.

Box 4.2 gives more information about the extent of health risks associated with central obesity:

Box 4.2: Waist circumference measurements

Waist circumference related to risks of metabolic complications of obesity			
Gender	Low (cm)	High (cm)	Very high (cm)
Male	Less than 94*	94 – 102	more than 102
Female	Less than 80	80 – 88	more than 88

* if measured in inches rather than centimetres then 94cms is ~ 37inches; 80cms is ~ 32inches; 102cms is ~ 40inches; 88cms is ~ 35inches

So what about your actual weight?

Are you really overweight/obese? What's your:	Body mass index (BMI)? =
	Waist circumference? =
	Waist: hips ratio? =

As we age, being overweight puts more stress on our joints and can make our mobility more difficult. Being very overweight (termed obese) is linked to higher rates of cancer that someone would not have developed if they had stayed slim. Cancers of the breast, ovary, uterus, prostate, pancreas and colon for instance are much more like to happen if someone is obese. As the years go by, women who are obese are twelve times more likely to develop diabetes, four times more likely to suffer from raised blood pressure, and three times more likely to have a heart attack.

As you get your weight down to normal levels, your risk of heart disease plummets to normal too, and hopefully your menopausal symptoms will also improve. There'll be lots of other health benefits, like reducing the likelihood of diabetes, or improving control of blood sugar levels if someone already has diabetes. Evidence shows that taking exercise and sticking to a healthy diet aids a person with asthma to gain better control of their symptoms such as being short of breath when they are out walking - even improving their asthma symptom score by 50%!

Fashionable diets involving liquid replacement meals or fasting may not be sustainable for more than a few days or weeks. You need to get into healthy eating habits to maintain the weight loss you manage to achieve – forever – during and after your menopause.

Apps & websites for supporting healthy eating and weight control - some takeaway healthy messages

To lose weight there are many approaches you can try to help you to improve your diet and sustain any weight loss:

NHS weight loss plan app: This app focusses on helping the user over the course of 12 weeks to focus on their weight and the goals they have set for themselves. The app helps you on your weight loss journey by helping you to record your food and drink intake, and activity levels. There are also some useful guides telling you about the benefits of embarking on this path, as well as tips about a healthy diet and how to calculate your BMI and much more.

The app encourages users to log their weight loss and waist size each week to see how they progress in their weight loss journey. The app is free, but the app will prompt you to agree to its terms and conditions, as well as confirming that you are over 18 years of age.

Use the **NHS BMI calculator** to check your body mass index (BMI) to find out if you need to lose weight, if you are underweight or you are at a healthy weight. This is a free tool to use but you need to input information such as your height, weight, age, sex, ethnicity and activity level.

https://www.nhs.uk/live-well/healthy-weight/bmi-calculator/

Calculate what your daily calorie intake should be using the NHS website. The amount of calories you are recommended to take will be unique to you, as it depends on your age (younger people generally need more calories than older people); your lifestyle (inactive people need less calories than active people); your size (your overall height and weight). Calories are a measure of how much energy your food or drink contain.

https://www.nhs.uk/common-health-questions/food-and-diet/what-should-my-daily-intake-of-calories-be/

Be more mindful in your eating. Track meals, habits and calories by recording what you eat each day accurately, using tracking apps such as *MyFitnessPal* and the *NHS food scanner*.

MyFitnessPal app/website: The *MyFitnessPal* app allows you to set your own calorie and nutrition goals based on your current weight, how much you wish to lose and your activity levels. The app allows you to track your food and activity whilst seeing the 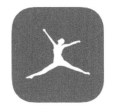 breakdown of each nutrient to guide your future dietary choices.

The app allows you to scan food items and record recipes for easy logging onto your personal diary. The blog feature allows you to see lots of exercise and dietary recommendations, as well as guide you to make plans and recipes to inspire you.

The app is free for the basic features but the app will prompt you to set up a free account using your email address. You can also upgrade to the premium version which gives you access to premium features such as more nutritional insights, but this comes at a cost.

https://www.myfitnesspal.com/

The NHS Food Scanner app: The app allows you to easily scan food items to see what they contain. The app offers food swap recommendations for healthier alternatives. The app is unique in the way that it shows you visually what your food contains, 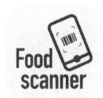 and allows you to see when you have made healthier choices.

The app is free, but the app will prompt you to sign up to its terms and conditions and give access to your camera on the device that you are using.

Staying active - keep going

Being active is beneficial to menopausal women in so many ways; yet so many women stop exercising at this time in their lives. The many benefits of physical exercise during, and after, the menopause include: helping women manage and cope with menopausal symptoms, improving their self-esteem and strengthening their bones. For many women the menopause also coincides with changes in their home lives, as if they have had children, their kids are often at the age when they are leaving home.

This is a great opportunity to invest in yourself. Try a new hobby, join a club or go walking with friends. Getting active is so easy – it really is! If you drive, park further away from the shops and walk there, or take the stairs rather than go up an escalator or in a lift. Ask for medical advice before you start exercising if you have any concerns or health problems about becoming more active.

A little activity is better than none. Keep on the move. Don't sit for long; get up and do something. Aim for walking at least 10,000 steps a day, every day – a target widely promoted for healthy living for all age groups. Start with less steps if you need to, then build up. Physical fitness becomes even more important the longer that you live.

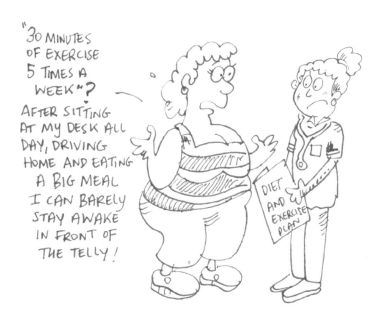

Find an exercise that suits you and that you enjoy. You are more likely to stick with it if you enjoy it. Get a pedometer to count how many steps that you do each day, or purchase a wrist monitor or smartwatch; although most mobile phones now can record your step count if you prefer that as your monitoring device. Wear it all day when you are walking to work, gardening or dancing.

You can monitor your heart rate when you are exercising - is that a feature of your smartwatch if you have one? If it is waterproof, you could use it whilst swimming or exercising in water too.

Apps and websites you can try to help you stay active

Couch to 5K app: This app, supported by the NHS, offers a free running plan for beginners with the aim of completing three runs a week to get you to running 5 kilometres (that's just over three miles) a day within nine weeks. Listen to audios during your runs to motivate you to make the active changes to your lifestyle and track your progress.

There are topics you can listen to, or read up on, to help you to achieve a healthier lifestyle including your mental wellbeing, adopting a healthy diet and how to join up with others in the community.

Couch to 5K allows you to choose a personal trainer to talk you through each run, and you can change this to different trainers along your journey if you prefer. The app gives you the option to state your sex and age to personalize your progress with the programme - but this is optional.

The app is free, but the app will prompt you to accept terms and conditions that note your location if you wish, as another option.

Emma (aged 60 years old) tells her story as to how the Couch to 5K app has helped her

"Throughout the menopause I found it really difficult to maintain a healthy lifestyle as sometimes I felt low in myself and did not have the energy to exercise or eat healthily. Once my menopausal symptoms became controlled I decided to get back into a healthier way of life. To help me to find the motivation I downloaded the Couch to 5K app. With the help of celebrity trainer Denise Lewis I felt able to take the steps I needed to become a healthier me. It was really sustainable and achievable as the transition to walking 5 kilometres a day was steady and I found myself becoming healthier and a better version of myself as the weeks went by, and they flew by! I felt inspired and ready to take control and change my lifestyle – which I've done and sustained now, four months later!"

Menopause and exercise free podcast:
This is a podcast by gynaecologist and founder of Menopause Magazine Dr Heather Currie who is joined by Jane Dowling from Meno and Me and Clare Taylor from Women in Sport. The podcast discusses menopause and exercise. The podcast content is free to access with no sign up needed. **The podcast is available at**:
https://audioboom.com/posts/7398601-menopause-and-exercise

NHS Active 10 Walking Tracker app: This app helps to motivate you to change your lifestyle by helping you to set targets and track how many minutes of brisk walking that you do. There are also articles giving advice about how to get back on track after taking a break, or walking after illness or injury.

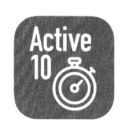

The app is free, but the app will prompt you to accept terms and conditions, enabling you to register to access the motion and fitness and location records of the walking that you do. The app gives you the option to state your sex and age too, for a more personalized review of the uptake of the programme - but again, this is optional.

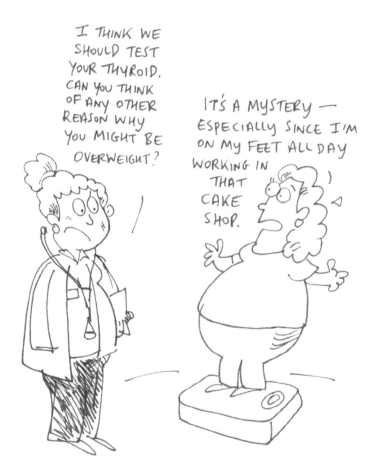

Sleep, glorious sleep

Many women experience some sleep disturbance during their menopause, even if they have never had sleeping problems before. Sleep patterns and the depth of sleep changes as we get older. It's normal for our sleep to be shorter, lighter and more fragmented as we age. However, poor sleep can really affect your quality of daily life. It can affect how you feel about yourself and others. When people don't get enough sleep, they often tend to snack more and consume more calories. 'Insomnia' is a term that describes poor quality sleep. That could be, difficulty getting off to sleep, staying asleep, or waking too early. What really matters is how fatigued you feel during the daytime, how much your concentration is impaired and how your mood is affected if you don't sleep.

Sleep may be disturbed by physical symptoms such as hot flushes, or emotional symptoms such as depression or anxiety. There are a number of actions that can help you to sleep better:

- Establish a 'bed time' routine that you follow every evening to prepare your body and mind for a peaceful night.
- Avoid nicotine, caffeine and alcohol in the late afternoon and evening. Most people can manage up to 400mg of caffeine a day; but more than 600mg a day has been linked to insomnia, irritability, raised blood pressure and more. Look at the specific caffeine content in high street coffees if you drink out – some are much stronger than others.
- Don't eat a large meal in the evening. Try having your main meal at lunchtime and a smaller meal in the evening.
- Try and avoid a nap in the daytime. Save your sleep for night time.
- Create a calm bedroom. Consider the colour of the walls, the textures of your bedding, the comfort of your mattress and pillows. If you are experiencing hot flushes, you may feel more comfortable layering your bedding and using natural fibres to keep you cool.

- Stay off your phone in the late evening and during the night – being engrossed in messages on your mobile phone and other devices can adversely affect your sleep.
- Reduce your stress levels; speak to your doctor if you think you are experiencing a low mood, anxiety or depression.
- Try meditation as part of your bedtime routine.

**Apps and websites that you can try to help you to improve your sleep
The Art of Restorative Sleep - The Happy Menopause Podcast**:
This podcast is by Lisa Cypers Kamen and she discusses why each stage of the sleep cycle is important and how to get a restorative night's sleep by improving your nutrition, lifestyle and more. The podcast content is free to access with no sign up needed.

https://www.well-well-well.co.uk/the-art-of-restorative-sleep-the-happy-menopause-podcast

Information about insomnia is on the NHS website: this includes how to know if you do have insomnia. There is also a sleep self-assessment chart where you can indicate if you do suffer from insomnia and the potential causes. The website content is free to access with no sign up needed.

https://www.nhs.uk/conditions/insomnia

Menopause and Sleep - The sleep charity website: This webpage explains how the menopause can affect your sleep and the link between the menopause and insomnia. There is further explanation about how to improve your sleep during the menopause with helpful advice and tips. The website content is free to access with no sign up needed.

https://thesleepcharity.org.uk/information-support/adults/sleep-hub/menopause-and-sleep

Enjoying sex – some like it hot!

Women during the menopause may feel differently about their bodies as they may experience changes in their feelings towards sex. Some women enjoy sex more, but many others do not. The vaginal area can become dry and painful leading to soreness and avoidance of sex. However, there are many 'over the counter' products that you can buy to try and relieve this problem - such as lubricants. Silicone and water based lubricants are safe to use with condoms; oil based lubricants can damage condoms.

Many women experience vaginal soreness despite using lubricants. Often this is due to generalized vaginal dryness and not simply during sex. Applying vaginal oestrogen gel will often help.

This can be prescribed by your doctor for most women, apart from some who have had specific breast cancer treatments, and should avoid it. It can also be bought over the counter. So, why not seek confidential help from your pharmacist or family doctor about this?

For other women there may be an underlying problem with dry skin, or they may not wish to use vaginal oestrogen. In these cases, natural oils such as olive oil, sweet almond oil, wheatgerm oil or coconut oil can be helpful. These oils however should not be used with condoms.

Even though you might not be menstruating, or your periods have become irregular, you may still be ovulating and therefore can become pregnant! You are best using contraception for two years after your last period if they have stopped before you are 50 years old, and use contraception for one year if your last period occurs after the age of 50 years old. If you do not want to become pregnant then choose a contraception to suit your needs. Some forms of hormonal contraception which contain progesterone only may mask the onset of your menopause by stopping your periods completely. These include the progesterone only pill (POP), the contraceptive implant or injection and the intrauterine system (Mirena, Mylena, Jaydesse). The combined oral contraceptive pill contains both oestrogen and progesterone, so while you may still have periods the oestrogen content might mask your menopause symptoms. It is best therefore to discuss with your GP or family planning nurse how and when to stop your contraception.

The National Menopause Association website: The website offers information about pregnancy and the menopause, when it may be possible to get pregnant, how to know if you are still fertile, how to increase your chances of getting pregnant and the potential risks. The website content is free to access with no sign up needed.

https://nationalmenopauseassociation.com/can-you-get-pregnant-during-menopause/

This is suitable for: perimenopause

Safe Sex: If you have different sexual partners or are starting a new sexual relationship, be aware of your risk of catching a sexually transmitted infection (STI). These are avoidable by using a condom; different types of condoms are available on the market.

Information about different types of condoms is available at:
https://www.health.com/condition/sexual-health/types-of-condoms

If you are concerned that you might have an STI, go for a check up at a sexual health clinic as soon as possible.

Information on sexually transmitted infections is available on the NHS website.
https://www.nhs.uk/conditions/sexually-transmitted-infections-stis/

Cervical smear changes during the menopause can make having a smear a different experience to how it felt before the menopause. See Jo's cervical cancer trust for tips on having a smear test after the menopause.

https://www.jostrust.org.uk/about-us/news-and-blog/smear-tests-after-menopause

This is suitable for: perimenopause, postmenopause, premature and surgical menopause

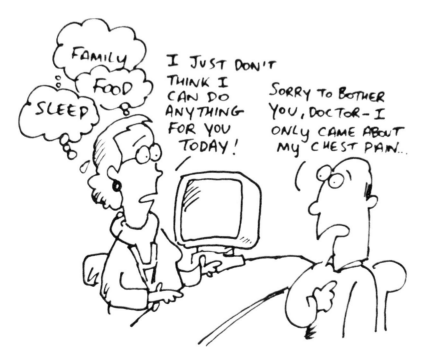

Menopause and the workplace – work at it

Nowadays, women are living longer than previously. Furthermore, most of us have careers spanning more decades which means that menopause in the workplace has become an issue that previous generations may not have experienced.

Unfortunately, despite the menopause workplace pledge most women find themselves unsupported in the workplace when it comes to help and respect for those experiencing menopausal symptoms. As such, many women over 50 years old go on to leave their work earlier than they would have wished, or reduce their hours, due to the symptoms that they are experiencing. It is thought that one in four women experiencing the menopause have considered leaving their job due to their symptoms. Without appropriate workplace support, women who are experiencing menopausal related symptoms such as hot flushes, poor memory, anxiety, fatigue may be less productive or be more likely to take time off work.

There is hope that women can cope better with their menopausal symptoms at work from adopting simple remedies and strategies, as well as a change in attitudes and enablement at an organisational level. The first step is to raise awareness of the facts around the menopause and its impact on someone's work. So, this is not just about raising awareness in women, but also to get the headlines to all staff, especially line managers who have responsibilities for sustaining the health and wellbeing of their staff. Women should not be discriminated against due to their menopausal state.

Workplace modifications such as fans, frequent breaks and access to water are essential. Lightweight uniforms, particularly in summer months are also helpful. A workplace menopause café, either face to face or online, is somewhere safe where women can share their experiences and tips with each other. Examples of this are hair care suggestions to use more natural hair products, avoiding tight ponytails which puts pressure on hair follicles, or changing to more natural skin products.

Menopausal support such as from a named menopause champion at work, or others at the menopause cafés can be facilitated by the organisation's human resources team, or occupational health staff, or by the women themselves. The main prerequisite is confidentiality, by providing a safe space to meet and talk, either virtually or face to face.

There are resources for encouraging employers to develop menopause policies to create more supportive environments where any stigma is addressed, there is more awareness of menopause issues, with help for women experiencing the menopause to stay and progress at work.
See the advice on the British Menopause Society, NHS, and wellbeing of women websites, to name but a few. The women's charity *Wellbeing of Women* has initiated an online pledge where both women and their employers can sign up to making positive changes in the workplace.

The Menopause support toolkit: This is a toolkit for employers to download for current guidance and resources to help people in their workplace who are going through the menopause. The toolkit includes facts, advice on how to implement the advice into the workplace and tips from a leading expert.

The website content is free to access but it will prompt you to enter your company name, job title, work email address and name, in order to download the toolkit.

https://info.peppyhealth.com/menopause-support-toolkit-download

Alcohol – sobering thoughts
Alcohol can make existing health conditions worse and change the way we behave, putting us at risk. Drinking in excess during the menopause may increase your risks of osteoporosis, type 2 diabetes, depression, cancer and weight gain. Alcoholic drinks are full of hidden calories. A pint of beer is nearly 200 calories and a 750ml bottle of wine is about 600 calories. As many as one in five adults drink an unhealthy amount of alcohol regularly.

Read more about these risks in the
Alcohol and Menopause: Things to Consider – My Menopause Magazine

https://www.mymenopausemag.com/menopause/alcohol-and-menopause-things-consider

Alcohol intake? Complete the Fast Alcohol Screening Test (FAST) questionnaire (see Box 4.3) to gauge how much alcohol you're really drinking, and when you see your score think if you should be concerned and take action. The minimum score is 0 and the maximum score is 16. A score of 3 onwards for any of the four questions may indicate that you are engaging in hazardous drinking. Listen to other people too if they tell you that they think you're drinking too much alcohol- they are probably right, and you could be in denial. If a doctor or nurse asks you how much alcohol you drink- tell them the truth- you want to be as healthy as possible don't you and get their realistic advice and support?

Box 4.3: FAST questionnaire

(1 drink = ½ pint beer or 1 glass wine or 1 single shot of spirits)

1. Men: How often do you have eight or more drinks on one occasion?
    Women: How often do you have six or more drinks on one occasion?
    never / less than monthly / monthly / weekly / daily or almost daily

2. How often during the last year have you been unable to remember what happened the night before because you had been drinking?
    never / less than monthly / monthly / weekly / daily or almost daily

3. How often during the last year have you failed to do what was normally expected of you because of drinking?
    never / less than monthly / monthly / weekly / daily or almost daily

4. In the last year has a relative or friend, or a doctor or other health worker been concerned about your drinking or suggested you cut down?
    no / yes on one occasion / yes more than one occasion

Scores:
Questions 1,2,3 score = 0, 1, 2, 3, 4 for the answers (e.g., 'never' = 0; 'daily or almost daily' = 4);
Question 4 score = 0, 2, 4 respectively

It's a good idea to keep a daily diary of how much you are drinking for about two weeks. Many people can underestimate their alcohol intake by as much as 40%. Alcohol content varies between drinks (based on the size of the drink and its alcohol strength), so be sure as to how many units of alcohol you are measuring. Units are a simple way of expressing the quantity of alcohol in a drink. National advice for women is to limit the amount of alcohol they drink to less than 14 units a week

https://www.nhs.uk/live-well/alcohol-advice/calculating-alcohol-units/

Many people who drink too much alcohol hide it from their friends, family and work colleagues.

So, if you feel that you drink too much, *own up to it!*

Try reducing your alcohol intake slowly, setting realistic targets. You might try having one drink-free day a week, then increase it to two alcohol-free days a week. Maybe you could meet friends in an alcohol free place or do some exercise instead of sitting in a bar or, set yourself a two drink limit. You may need to change your lifestyle a bit to beat the issue and avoid temptations.

Try keeping a daily log of the amount of alcohol you drink using the table below and review it at the end of the week. Be honest about what you drink...your log is there to help you.

Table 4.1: A typical week's diary logging your alcohol intake (honestly!)							
	Monday	Tuesday	Wednesday	Thursday	Friday	Saturday	Sunday
Drinks							
Units							
Calories							

Online information on the risks of drinking excessive alcohol and need to quit

Using the NHS Drink free days app should help you to feel healthier, lose weight and save money. Just pick your days to skip alcohol and get practical support to stick with it.

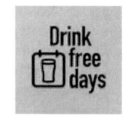

DrinkCoach app: This app allows you to monitor your alcohol consumption, calorie intake and the amount of money that you spend on alcohol. You can set notes to motivate yourself and stay on track towards meeting your goals. The event diary records

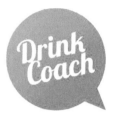

hangovers, arguments and accidents to allow you to understand how drinking too much alcohol may affect you - and you can then reflect on those findings.

The *DrinkCoach* app is unique in the way that it is personalised to match what you actually drink. It allows you to use the tracker and look at how you are progressing towards your goals. Mindfulness videos within the app can help you to manage your cravings. The app is free for access to, and use of, the basic features. You can also upgrade to book online appointments for a fixed price to discuss your drinking and receive guidance in a confidential environment.

Investing in yourself by self-care; it's in your best interests
Each woman's journey through the menopause is individual. Some women feel a sense of freedom with the menopause. For other women though this can be a really difficult time in their lives. For those women who feel like 'empty nesters' when their children leave their home, they can feel lonely, isolated and experience grief.

What is shared however for all women, is the benefit we feel when we take care of ourselves. It is vital that as we age and transition through the menopause, we accept our bodily changes will happen, and embrace a 'new you'.

Changes in your hormone levels can impact on both your mental health and physical health. You may experience anxiety, depression, anger, frustration, low self-esteem and poor concentration ('brain fog').

There are several resources that you can connect to for advice and help:

Menopause Matters website: This website looks at a wide variety of topics surrounding the menopause such as menopause in the workplace, treatments and therapies such as HRT, and how to access health professionals to talk to.

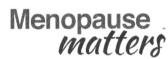

Menopause Matters also allows you to talk to other women in the community within forums to discuss current topics. The website content is free to access with no sign up needed, however you can sign up for free using your email address for a free newsletter.

https://www.menopausematters.co.uk/

Suitable for: perimenopause, postmenopause, premature and surgical menopause

Daisy Network website: The website looks specifically at premature ovarian insufficiency and explores the diagnositic process, the signs and symptoms and links to current research being explored for the condition. The Daisy Network is a charity. The basic website content is free to access with no sign up needed;

however you can become a member for a fixed cost each year to allow you to be a part of a Daisy Network Facebook group, with other members and free online counselling for premature ovarian insufficiency.

https://www.daisynetwork.org/

Suitable for: premature menopause

Leah (aged 37 years old) felt really supported in combating the effects of her menopause by looking and learning from the Daisy Network website

"As a young woman I found it really difficult to find any information about the menopause for women in my age group. I felt alone and that nobody else was going through the same thing as me, and it was incredibly isolating to be so unsupported. This all changed when a friend recommended the Daisy Network organisation. Once I found their website I understood my diagnosis of premature ovarian insufficiency better, and realised that there are many women worldwide who are going through the same thing as me. My signs and symptoms then made sense and I was then able to read up on the range of HRT resources available, so I could move forwards in a way that was best for me. I felt so much more supported and uplifted after finding the Daisy Network, as I am able to keep up to date with new ongoing research into my condition."

Menopause Cafés: Menopause Cafés can give women the opportunity to meet in locations across the UK and in other countries to discuss the menopause in a confidential space, which is open for all. There is an events calendar on the website showing all the upcoming café locations and other events on a larger scale such as the annual festivals. The website content and Menopause Cafés are free to access but they do offer the chance to make donations.

https://www.menopausecafe.net

'Queermenopause' website: This website focusses on those who identify in the LGBTQ+ community and it discusses menopause for those in these groups, with links to useful resources and podcasts to further their understanding. The website also looks at the portrayal of the 'Queer Menopause' in the media and research that is being undertaken. The website content is free to access.

https://www.queermenopause.com

The NHS Inform website: This website describes different types of talking therapies to help you to think in a more positive way. This is about training yourself to recognise behaviours and thoughts that hold you back and respond more positively. Cognitive behavioural therapy (CBT) can help by breaking down the cluster of problems that seem to be leading to your stressed state, into five areas: thoughts, feelings, physical symptoms, behaviour and environmental factors.

Counselling is another type of 'talking therapy', available through your family doctor, occupational health or other health services. It can help you through issues or concerns that affect your mental health. The website describes all of these therapies and which is suitable for each person. The website content is free to access.

https://www.nhsinform.scot/healthy-living/mental-wellbeing/therapy-and-counselling/talking-therapies-explained

Psychological wellbeing – you know the risks so, mind out

For some women, the psychological impact of the menopause can be disruptive and affect their mental health. There are various treatment options that might help to relieve some of the psychological impacts of the menopause. It is important to look after yourself physically too. Eating a healthy diet, exercising regularly and mindfulness can help.

Maximise your use of digital aids like the apps scattered through this book, and other equipment and devices that are accessible and available that can support you in achieving this positive behaviour change.

So, assess how ready you are to change your lifestyle habits and way of life, and ensure that you try to stay fit and mobile, overcome any menopause related issues such as sweats or low mood – and plot and access the range of help and assistive technology resources you'll need.

You must motivate yourself to optimise your health and wellbeing by harnessing your friends' and family's support, resisting temptations, and finding satisfaction in your everyday life - with consistently healthy habits.

To improve your lifestyle and sustain all these positive benefits long-term means that you must want to change, then progress to preparing to change, and move on to actually making those changes. You may relapse and need encouragement to then repeat the process and sustain the changes you've made to your everyday life and behaviour. So, take a look and work through the five stages of the cycle of change below to think through and plan what you need to do to overcome any problems in accomplishing your healthy lifestyle goals, and try to stick with your achievements forever.

So off you go......begin to build your action plan to identify your resource needs to lead a happy, safe and independent life; describing where you are now, what your goals are, how you are going to reach those goals and sustain your improved life.

I'm not obese doctor – I've just got slow metabolism

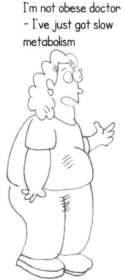

Never mind your metabolism - it's your walking speed that needs to improve. It will help you combat your menopausal symptoms.

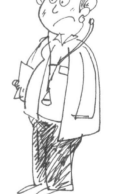

Your five stages of change – take the heat off your daily life

1. ***Pre-contemplation***: you've no intention to change your behaviour in the foreseeable future.

So even if you are overweight, or sitting down for most of the day, or just about managing in your everyday life…..you're oblivious to any risks or don't really care……..or don't see the benefits………

So now describe your current thinking about the life you're living, if you're oblivious or are not particularly bothered about the state of your daily life or independence or health and wellbeing such as your menopausal symptoms:

2. *Contemplation*: you are aware of the problems that exist and are seriously thinking about overcoming them but have not yet made a commitment to take action.

So you're thinking of what changes you might take to your lifestyle and daily living....maybe reading or hearing good stories of how other people have made successful changes to their lives in overcoming menopause related suffering, that you could mirror?

So now describe your current thinking about any problems that you are aware of in your daily life or independence or health and wellbeing, what changes you would like to make, and how and when that might be:

3. ***Preparation***: you are intending to take action in the next few days or months and (may) have unsuccessfully taken action in the past year.

So get ready…..steady……go. You've read this book avidly, absorbing all the useful information in each chapter that relates to you - such as the apps that might help you, the answers to the questions that you had too and the successful case studies throughout. So now think out what changes you'll make to your everyday living and home or work environment, and what assistive aids you'll need to buy (desk fan?), and what skills you'll need to be more confident to use digital aids like apps and personal assistants, and assistive devices for your daily life; or what groups you might join.

So now describe what actions you plan to take and changes that you hope to make in relation to the state of your daily life or your health and wellbeing – what/when/how, and describe what you will need to buy or access or learn too:

4. Action: you are now modifying your behaviour, experiences, or environment (including devices you now have access to) in order to overcome your weaknesses, and build these changes into your daily life with obvious benefits to your health and wellbeing and overcoming menopause-related symptoms and barriers.

So now describe the actions you have taken to improve the life you're living, and boost your health and wellbeing (be as specific as you can, describing how confident you now are in using digital aids like apps or accessing websites, listening to podcasts, talking through your problems at work with your line manager etc.):

5. *Maintenance*: you are working hard so as not to relapse; you're consolidating the gains you've attained

So now describe the actions you have taken to sustain your improved lifestyle and habits that boost your health and wellbeing to minimise the effects of the menopause (be as specific as you can, describing your use of digital aids like apps or behaviour changes). What further developments are you adopting or planning to maintain the positive changes to your lifestyle and habits – what/why/ when/how?

Keep it up!!

Doctors' insights

Isabelle (48 years old) presented with weight gain, mood swings, hot flushes, poor sleep and loss of libido. Her last period was nine months ago. Her Dad had a DVT (deep vein thrombosis) – a clot in his leg, her BMI was 33 showing that she was very overweight and her blood pressure was stable. She was very keen to start taking HRT and was prescribed a combined HRT patch (as this has a low side effect profile compared with oral hormone tablets) which soon helped with her symptoms.

Doctor's insights: topical HRT applied via the skin, can be used in patients with a family history of clots or cancers as side effects are relatively low when compared to the possible effects of oral HRT medications.

Dana (56 years old) who had a hysterectomy for heavy bleeding seven years ago, has been on oestrogen-only HRT since then. She went for an HRT review with the practice nurse. On examination her BP (blood pressure) was raised and her BMI (body mass index) was 40, which means she was classed as 'obese'. She had gained weight over the last few years. On discussion, her menopausal symptoms were much better, and so she agreed to take a lower dose of oestrogen tablets, as oestrogen can trigger weight gain and also can affect someone's BP.

Doctor's insights: you don't need to take HRT as a lifelong treatment. You can stop it, or take a lower dose and stop eventually. The longer you take the HRT, the more prone you are to get related side effects.

Chapter 5 Clinical management of the menopause

Hormone replacement therapy; the prescription for change

Hormone replacement therapy (HRT) consists of hormones - oestrogen, progesterone or testosterone, used to treat menopausal symptoms. Oestrogen is the hormone that helps to combat menopausal symptoms. However, oestrogen alone can cause changes in the cells lining the womb leading to cancer in some cases. To minimise this, progesterone can be prescribed as well.

If more than a year has passed since a woman has had her last period, she can have continuous 'combined' or 'no bleed' HRT. This is where oestrogen and progesterone are prescribed to be taken every day. If less than a year has passed since her last period, or if the woman is still having periods, she will be prescribed 'cyclical' HRT. In this form she will take oestrogen every day, along with progesterone for 12-14 days of her monthly cycle.

If a woman wishes to have 'no bleed' HRT but is still having periods there is only one option. That is to have oestrogen as a patch, gel or spray along with a Mirena coil or, intrauterine system (IUS) to provide progesterone. In this case the progesterone in the IUS is released continuously, resulting in a 'no bleed' form of HRT.

HRT comes in various forms depending on the woman's medical history and her needs. There are patches, gels, sprays, oral tablets, vaginal tablets, or creams as well as the IUS:

- Oestrogen: tablet to be taken orally; or transdermal (applied directly to the skin) in the form of a patch, gel or spray; or vaginal as cream, tablet, ring, or pessary
- Progesterone: tablet (micronised progesterone, progestins); or via an intrauterine system (IUS)
- Oestrogen & progesterone combined: as a patch or tablet
- Testosterone: as gel or pump

In general, the transdermal patches, gels or sprays along with the progesterone tablet or IUS are considered the safest options. The preferred choice will depend on what suits the individual woman's preferences and needs, and her personal medical history.

The British Menopause Society offers information and advice on HRT on their website:

https://thebms.org.uk

Good news for women living in England is that they can access a year's worth of HRT for the cost of two prescriptions, currently £18.70 (if they do not have exemption for a health or other reason from paying for their medication). The woman must take out a pre-payment certificate (PPC), which will be available at a pharmacy registered to sell PPCs. The certificate will be valid for twelve months and cover an unlimited number of HRT items such as patches, tablets and topical preparations – so long as they are on the approved long list of HRT medications.

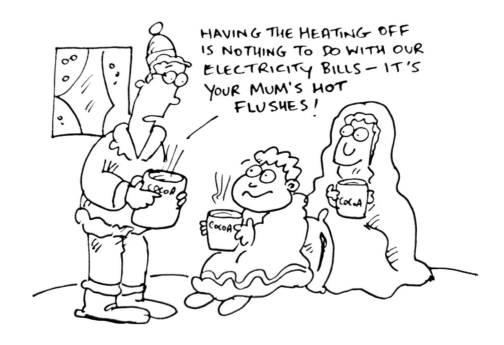

Benefits of HRT – hot news
Like all drugs, the range of HRT treatments have benefits and risks. The main benefit of HRT is in relieving menopausal symptoms – hot flushes, night sweats and mood changes which can start to improve within a few days of starting HRT medication. Other symptoms like vaginal dryness or musculoskeletal pains can take a few weeks to start to improve. Treating hot flushes and night-time sweats (vasomotor symptoms) leads to improved sleep and energy levels. There is also an improvement in brain fog, concentration, and memory (cognitive symptoms) which in turn help to improve the woman's work related performance. HRT also helps to reduce muscular aches and pains allowing women to exercise more comfortably. This in turn helps with their weight control and overall wellbeing.

HRT also helps a woman's sexual function by treating oestrogen deficiency and improving their wellbeing. Testosterone can also be used to treat reduced sexual desire due to the menopause where HRT alone has not helped.

HRT improves bone strength and so helps to prevent osteoporosis. This in turn reduces a person's risk of fractures (breaks) caused by osteoporosis.

HRT also reduces a woman's risk of heart disease. This is the case where HRT is started before the age of 60 years old, or within 10 years of the menopause. It is important however to ensure that any existing heart conditions are treated as well. HRT alone is not a treatment for heart disease.

Risks of HRT – cutting down
HRT does have risks depending on the health condition in question, the type of HRT and the woman's age. There are many misconceptions about the dangers of HRT; for most women the benefits of HRT usually outweigh the small risks. Women who take combined oestrogen and progesterone HRT have a slight increase in breast cancer. This amounts to 10 extra cases of breast cancer for every 1000 women aged 50-59 years old who take oestrogen and progesterone HRT for five years.

While there is an increased chance of getting breast cancer, the risk of dying from the disease is not increased, if it is spotted and treated.

It is also important to remember that women who are obese and who drink excess alcohol (> 14 units per week) have a similarly increased risk of breast cancer. If they then have HRT as well, their overall risk is increased further. If having considered all options it is felt that they do need HRT, the gels, patches, or sprays with micronized progesterone or a Mirena coil are the safest options. Women who have had a hysterectomy (their womb has been surgically removed) and who have oestrogen - only HRT have very little, or no, increased risk of breast cancer.

Furthermore, vaginal oestrogen does not increase the risk of a woman getting breast or womb cancer. This is because it comes as a very low dose and does not get absorbed into the bloodstream by this vaginal route.

Blood clots, thrombosis or stroke can be another risk of taking HRT. These risks are increased in women who are obese, or are smokers, and who have underlying medical conditions. Again, the risks are greater if women have both oestrogen and progesterone and if they have it in combination tablet form. Oestrogen only HRT does not increase the risk of having a blood clot or stroke.

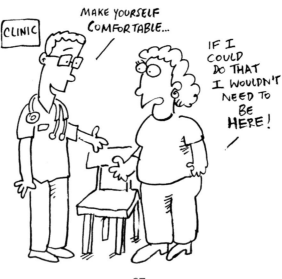

Duration of HRT treatment – as long as you need it

There is no cut off time limit for taking HRT. However, at present the benefits in prevention of heart disease do not seem to extend beyond the age of 60 years. After this, we know that the risks of breast cancer, stroke and blood clots increase. At this point most women will have a discussion with their doctor weighing the risks versus the benefits of continuing their HRT. This discussion needs to consider the woman's personal risks as well as the type of HRT she is taking and her other lifestyle factors.

If a woman decides to stop HRT, her symptoms are likely to return. She may gradually reduce, or suddenly stop the HRT, but this will make no difference as to whether her symptoms return. Overall, it is felt that for most women the benefits they experience from HRT far outweigh the risks involved.

If a woman has been on HRT into her 60s or beyond and stops, but wishes to restart because her symptoms have returned, a discussion around the risks and benefits for her must take place with the clinician who prescribed her HRT medication. If on the other hand a woman wants to start HRT for the first time in later life the risks of HRT are far greater than if she had taken HRT previously.

Contraception and the menopause – do what you conceive to be right

It is important to remember that HRT is not a contraceptive and so does not prevent unwanted pregnancy. The only exception is where the IUS (Mirena coil) is used to provide the progesterone component of a woman's HRT (but might also serve as a contraceptive too). At present, women under the age of 50 years should use contraception for two years after their last period. After the age of 50 years contraception is advised for one year after the last period. Overall, it is felt that contraception can be discontinued after the age of 55 years whether a woman is still experiencing periods, or hormone related bleeds, or not.

Sexually Transmitted Infections (STIs) – avoid, avoid, avoid

While STIs are uncommon in menopausal women it is still possible to catch an infection. Women should therefore ensure that they use condoms in any new sexual relationships. They should also get tested for STIs if they develop symptoms such as discharge, bleeding or pain, or if they consider themselves at risk.

Bleeding from HRT

Bleeding in the first three months of taking HRT is a common side effect of taking combined (oestrogen & progesterone) HRT. This may be any bleeding at all when taking a no-bleed preparation, or irregular bleed with cyclical HRT. This usually settles within three months. If it doesn't settle then changing the brand or type of HRT will often help; for example, switching from patches to a gel and progesterone tablet. Alternatively, it might be necessary to alter the dose, increasing the progesterone or decreasing the oestrogen components.

If bleeding continues after six months in spite of modifying the HRT then other causes of bleeding must be looked for. A full history and examination looking at risk factors for cancer of the cervix or womb should be carried out.

Investigations such as a pelvic ultrasound or taking a biopsy from the lining of the womb are sometimes needed. HRT is usually discontinued while investigations are being carried out. On some occasions it is then advised to insert an IUS (Mirena coil) to help thin out the lining of the womb and thus prevent further bleeding.

Testosterone maybe

Levels of testosterone and loss of libido are not directly related as female sexual desire is affected by several other factors including: relationships, social, domestic and health status. These issues as well as background oestrogen deficiency should be addressed prior to adding testosterone to a woman's HRT regime.

Testosterone is not currently licensed for prescribing for use in women in the United Kingdom. In practice, testosterone is prescribed off licence for treating low sexual desire for women where HRT alone has not been effective. But it should only be prescribed with advice or support from an expert or specialist.

Testosterone levels should be checked prior to treatment and every year during treatment. This is to ensure that the levels remain in the normal female range and to minimise the risk of side effects such as acne, excess male pattern hair growth, baldness and weight gain.

HRT and endometriosis; a complicated issue

Endometriosis is where cells from the lining of the womb are found in other parts of the pelvis. These cells bleed every month and cause pelvic pain, pain on intercourse and sometimes fertility problems. Treatment may involve inducing the menopause with medication or having surgery to remove a woman's ovaries and womb.

Women who undergo these treatments are often younger and will need HRT for protection against osteoporosis and heart disease. Adding HRT until the age of their natural menopause does not increase their risks of getting breast cancer. These younger women often require higher doses of oestrogen than women who have a natural menopause. Some also experience a more dramatic loss of libido, particularly with a surgically induced menopause.

In this situation, even though the womb is removed it is usual to have combined oestrogen and progesterone HRT initially. This is to reduce the risk of pelvic pain and, to reduce the very small risk of developing a cancer in any remaining endometriosis cells.

Allied medication – get help when you need it

Some other medication might be prescribed as well as, or instead of, HRT – depending on how well HRT as an entity controls a woman's menopausal symptoms.

Vaginal moisturisers and/or lubricants or low-dose vaginal oestrogen can be useful for urogenital symptoms like vaginal dryness.

Tibolone (brand name livial) can be prescribed as a short-term treatment that is similar to taking combined HRT (that is, oestrogen plus progesterone). It can help to relieve symptoms such as hot flushes, reduced sex drive and low mood – for postmenopausal women.

It might be that a person with a low mood might benefit from anti-depressant medication. Cognitive behavioural therapy (CBT) might help too alongside an anti-depressant drug – see Chapter 6 for more information about alternative therapies like these.

Clonidine is a prescription medicine used to lower blood pressure; but it can be prescribed to help to reduce a woman's hot flushes and night sweats.

Gabapentin is generally prescribed for epilepsy and other seizure disorders; but it can help to combat menopausal symptoms like hot flushes; though it is not currently licensed for this usage in the UK.

Doctors' insights

Barbara (47 years old) who had had a hysterectomy for cervical cancer in the recent past presented with menopausal symptoms. She was taking sertraline (an anti-depressant medication) for her low mood related symptoms, along with trialling an oestrogen patch.

Doctor's insights: as she was still having menopausal symptoms we swapped her treatment to try topical oestradiol gel (applied to her skin) and also changed her type of anti-depressant to venlafaxine. Two months later, she is doing much better with the changes made. So - hormone patches don't suit all women with menopausal symptoms, and their responsible clinician should consider alternative topical or oral treatment.

Christine (50 years old) presented with symptoms of anxiety, sleeplessness, tiredness for seven days prior to her periods every month. Her symptoms got better when her periods were over.
She tried various anti-depressants like sertraline and then citalopram for a good few months, with little effect. Hence, she was referred to the PMS (pre-menstrual syndrome) clinic at her local hospital. She was seen by a specialist in premenstrual exacerbation of psychological symptoms. When she was asked to fill in the symptom chart - she described her symptoms as fitting in every category, but they diminished after her periods ended. This is not a typical description of PMS, although she had premenstrual exacerbation. As her periods were heavy and irregular, the gynaecology specialist decided to do an endometrial biopsy and insert a Mirena coil providing progesterone, at the same time. Once the Mirena coil was in place she had an oestrogen patch – so that the combination of oestrogen and progesterone medication would help her symptoms.

Doctor's insights: some patients need further investigations or specialist input before starting the right HRT that suits their personal condition.

Eileen (58 years old) had had a hysterectomy and was still struggling with menopausal symptoms. She was using 25mcg oestrogen patches but wanted to increase the dose. She had a strong family history of breast cancer – her niece, and sister both developed breast cancer in their 40s. Her GP explained the risks of taking HRT guiding her through a scientific table from a reliable source, brought up on display on the computer screen. Eileen became fully aware of the risks involved but declined to consider any alternative and was willing to take risks involved with continuing to take 'oestrogen only' HRT.

Doctor's insights: all patients should be allowed to balance their risks of taking medication or not, and enabled to make an informed decision that suits them.

Fiona (41 years old) had had a hysterectomy for adenomyosis and endometriosis, had severe menopausal symptoms – including hot flushes, mood swings and sweats very much affecting her quality of life. She had a family history of thromboembolism (blood clots). She was very slim, a regular runner and a non-smoker. She was advised by her gynaecologist specialist to take combined HRT containing oestrogen and progesterone for six months to combat her endometriosis, and to continue her HRT treatment until she reached the average age of the menopause.

Doctor's insights: yes, even after a hysterectomy a woman may need to take combined HRT to continue to treat other conditions like endometriosis.

Helen (55 years old) had been on HRT for the last seven months. She had started to bleed but was not keen to stop taking HRT. Her body mass index (BMI) showed that she was very overweight with a BMI of 37, and she suffered from a raised blood pressure (hypertension) and diabetes. She had no known family history of cancer. Her GP was concerned about her bleeding and arranged an abdominal scan to check her endometrial thickness (lining of her uterus) which turned out to be 8.5mm – much thicker than expected for her age. So, her GP wrote to a gynaecologist to ask for advice. The specialist wanted to see Helen to organise a hysteroscopy, endometrial biopsy and consider the insertion of a Mirena coil. Unfortunately, the biopsy showed early signs of uterine cancer.

Doctor's insights: sometimes bleeding in a woman taking HRT warrants further investigations.

Chapter 6
Complementary and alternative treatments
for management of menopause

During the menopause, your body is producing less oestrogen which can result in you experiencing many physical or psychological symptoms. For some women, these symptoms may be a mild nuisance that doesn't affect their day-to-day life. However, for other women, these symptoms affect them so significantly, that they find their 'usual' activities (for example working in their job) become more challenging. The good news is that ... the menopause doesn't last forever. But, increasingly there are a range of complementary and other non-clinical therapies that can help you along your menopause journey. These may bring relief to both your physical and psychological symptoms.

It is always a good idea to make sure that any health or wellbeing professional or therapist whom you visit, is registered and qualified. The Complementary and Natural Healthcare Council has a 'Find a Practitioner' section on their website:

https://www.cnhc.org.uk

The British Register of Complementary Practitioners has helpful information too.

https://brcp.uk

Complementary therapists have moved away from initiating pharmaceutical treatments and use natural approaches or remedies instead. There are many types of complementary therapies available and we have listed some of them here:
- Aromatherapy
- Colon hydrotherapy
- Healing
- Hypnotherapy
- Kinesiology

- Massage
- Acupuncture
- Naturopathy
- Black cohosh
- Nutritional therapy
- Reflexology
- Reiki
- Shiatsu
- Sports massage
- Sports therapy
- Tai Chi
- Yoga

Most of the information about the benefits of these therapies in helping troublesome menopausal symptoms are from anecdotal reports from users or therapists, and are not based on scientific research.

Complementary and alternative therapies are used for all sorts of common health conditions like depression, pain, gut problems; as well as for menopausal related symptoms. So, you might try different forms of therapy such as relaxation, acupuncture, meditation, yoga and then find one that suits you and your personal needs and preferences.

Acupuncture – key points
Acupuncture might help to alleviate some menopausal symptoms including night sweats, mood swings and altered sleep patterns – but a recent academic review found no significant evidence of benefits. Acupuncture points around the body are believed to, when stimulated, support a person's physical and emotional wellbeing.

Very thin sterile needles are inserted by the acupuncturist in specific areas of your body, into the skin and underlying tissues for therapeutic or preventative purposes. Instead of needle insertion, other methods can be used to stimulate your body's acupuncture points such as acupressure or laser light therapy. Side effects from acupuncture are uncommon.

If they do occur, you may get a slight itching around the site of the acupuncture or mild bruising. Your therapist can advise you further on this.

Reflexology, quite a 'feat'

Pressure is applied to areas of your feet (commonly) or your hand or your ear. The pressure applied to specific points stimulates various parts of the body. It is relaxing and is thought to have many benefits including reducing the frequency or severity of headaches, eliminating toxins from your body and boosting your metabolism. Reflexology aims to improve the functioning inside of your body such as within your organs and systems (digestive system, nervous system, circulatory system etc.).

Reflexology has been reported to be useful in relieving common menopausal symptoms such as hot flushes, sleep disruption, night sweats and feeling low in mood. Reflexology is non-invasive, in that, nothing actually enters your body. Some people have reported feeling lightheaded afterwards and having sore feet (if pressure was applied to their feet).

Cognitive Behavioural Therapy (CBT), think it through

This type of 'talking therapy' helps you to think in more positive ways. CBT is an effective option for improving hot flushes, night sweats and other menopausal symptoms – for any woman, whether or not they are taking prescribed HRT.

Cognitive behaviour therapy includes traditional cognitive behavioural approaches such as:
- self-monitoring e.g. keeping a diary of food eaten and the calorie and /or fat content; or how well your night sweats are controlled by the personal actions you take
- stimulus control – developing strategies to reduce your exposure to stimuli which may trigger you restarting inappropriate unhealthy eating and gorging treats
- coping with cravings
- stress management e.g. for stress induced, work pressures

- relaxation techniques
- learned self-control – breaking your cycle between certain stimuli to eating particular foods and eating inappropriately
- problem solving skills
- becoming fitter – setting behavioural goals, reflecting changes in your eating pattern or exercise habits
- mood management
- managing your work and family pressures better
- relapse prevention – various mechanisms so that you accept that lapses are to be expected and how you might avoid a 'relapse'
- avoiding self-defeating thinking e.g. 'all or nothing' thinking
- improving your body image.

See the guide *Talking therapies explained*, This is about training yourself to recognise what behaviours and thoughts that you have that hold you back, and respond in more positive ways. CBT helps by breaking down the cluster of problems leading to your stressed state into five areas: thoughts, feelings, physical symptoms, behaviour and environmental factors. So, these are all the sort of menopausal effects that many women experience.

Counselling is another type of 'talking therapy', available through your family doctor team, occupational health or through provider services. It can help you through the issues or concerns that affect your mental health.

https://www.nhsinform.scot/healthy-living/mental-wellbeing/therapy-and-counselling/talking-therapies-explained

Practising mindfulness in the menopause – mind out, cheer up

Mindfulness is an approach you can try to lift your mood, by focusing on your thoughts and feelings. There is some evidence to suggest that practising mind-body techniques can reduce symptoms such as hot flushes, body aches and increase your feeling of wellness.

You could try eating mindfully, if you want to regain a healthy weight. That means that you will envisage food before it's in front of you, then look at it. Next think how you'll enjoy it, then savour each mouthful, appreciate the after taste, reflect on the flavour and what was great about the food you've just eaten – then start again.

Everyone's different. You need your own personal approach - find and do whatever works for you. Mindfulness can be achieved through a variety of approaches including meditation and Tai Chi:

Meditation: can help you to improve your sleep, reduce your stress and anxiety levels, and sometimes reduce your hot flushes. It is important to practise meditation on a regular basis e.g. everyday to gain a focus, and increase your skills relating to this method of self-care.

Tai Chi: this form of exercise appears to generate mental and physical benefits for your body. In most regions of the UK you can access Tai Chi classes in local village halls, sports clubs or schools.

Online classes are also available, for example at the Tai Chi Foundation website. They offer both free and paid classes for a range of abilities. The website features some free recordings of prior sessions that you can watch at your leisure. You can register for future sessions (both free or paid sessions) by entering your email address. (Please note that fees for paid sessions are displayed in US dollars.)

https://www.taichifoundation.org/live-online-courses

There are some YouTube Tai Chi videos that are free to access; an example is the *Shaolin Qigong 15 Minute Daily Routine*.
Take a look at YouTube:
https://www.youtube.com/watch?v=y2RAEnWreoE

Yoga: boost your mind, body and spirit

Different kinds of yoga are focused on breathing and tranquillity.
The thinking is that the body and mind cannot function fully if air is not exchanged in the lungs in a proper way. Some yoga movements are gentle whilst others are physically demanding. Doing yoga sounds lazy, but it really stretches your muscles. Some focus on physical postures, whilst others push you to control your breathing and adopt meditation. It's likely that there are many yoga classes you can attend locally, but you can also access yoga online too – see the Menopause Yoga website.

Menopause Yoga is an adapted form of yoga focusing on the main symptoms of the menopause, using breathing techniques and meditation exercises. One-to-one sessions are available (see costs on the website) where you can have a consultation and work up a personalised plan. Online group sessions on Zoom are available, where you book via the website.

https://www.menopause-yoga.com

Now….take a look at how Julie managed to calm her nerves using yoga, moving from a fight or flight state of mind…………. to rest and digest.

Julie (52years old) is married with two teenage children, at the peak of her career, and caring for her ageing parents. She had no time for exercise, with a stressful job, and running around after family.
She drank too much alcohol and grabbed mainly junk food when she could too. Her main menopausal symptoms were hot flushes, brain fog, and insomnia.
Julie was so busy that feeling stressed had become her 'norm'.
Up early, checking emails on the way to the shower - a multi-tasking superstar. She tried joining a yoga class when the menopause hit. Insomnia meant she was usually awake as early as 3.30am as she feared arriving at work because she knew she would have a hot flush and found it so embarrassing.
And guess what? Practising yoga really helped her to relax as she used the breathing and meditation techniques she was taught. That gave her the determination to adopt a healthy lifestyle and organise her everyday life much better so that she coped well with all the pressures on her from family and work.

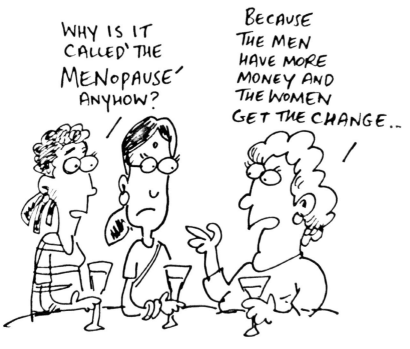

Herbal therapies maybe?

Herbal therapies such as St John's wort could improve your hot flushes and potentially depression too, associated with the menopause. Red clover is thought by some to help to minimise the frequency of hot flushes too, and could be worth trying. There is some evidence that hot flushes can be reduced by black cohosh – but do note that although the risk is rare, black cohosh has been associated with deteriorating liver function in one in 1000 – 10,000 women who try it for their menopause.

Evening primrose oil is a herbal remedy marketed as a dietary supplement in many countries. But although it has been trialled to overcome and treat postmenopausal symptoms, the latest clinical trials show little evidence of its benefits or effectiveness for the menopause.

Another widely recognised treatment for which there is little evidence that it is effective, is bioidentical hormone replacement therapy. The inventor claims that it can effectively treat the menopause, perimenopause and premenstrual, low libido, and erectile incontinence; but recent scientific evidence refutes this and confirms that there is no sound evidence to show that this therapy is effective for any of these conditions. Bioidentical hormones are unregulated 'natural' plant-derived combinations of hormones that are promoted as being similar or identical to human hormones. They are not licensed by UK regulatory bodies and so data regarding how effective they are, their purity, safety and side effects is unavailable or invalid.

Self-care – are you flush (lots of hormones not £s!)?

There are many practical actions you can take to help you to combat menopausal symptoms yourself. For instance, wear lighter clothing, use a fan at your work desk, keep your bedroom cool whilst you sleep, take a cool shower, adopt healthy lifestyle habits, avoid spicy foods and try to destress. Take a look at the range of symptoms that women can experience from the menopause in Chapter 9; then start finalising your action plan!

Doctor's insights

Anna (47 years old) went to see her GP as she had been struggling with tiredness for a while. Her last period was two years ago. She was not very keen on taking HRT as her mum had had breast cancer in her mid-fifties, and her mother believed that she might not have had that cancer if she'd not taken HRT for five years. Anna had her blood tested and was found to have very low iron levels, and a slightly low vitamin D level. She was keen to try alternative medication or another treatment rather than HRT. She discussed lifestyle modifications with her GP and got her friends' ideas too, drawn from their experiences. She decided to take iron and vitamin D supplements. She planned to increase her exercise and take regular walks with her partner.

Doctor's insights: So, not everyone is keen on HRT! HRT is not suitable for everyone and there are alternatives you can try like yoga and Tai Chi!!

Chapter 7 Top Tips

What to expect from a Women's Health Clinic – could be right up your street?

First step – make an appointment with a clinician at your general practice (could be your GP or practice nurse) to discuss what extra help a women's health clinic might offer you and if there is access to one nearby for you.

Do not self-diagnose the symptoms that you are having by using an internet search engine – it might mislead you and not recognise the real reason for what you are experiencing, and that might delay the diagnosis of a related serious health condition. Or it might be that you are making too much of your symptoms and get misled into trying menopausal treatments when actually you're not at the early or perimenopause stage yet.

It's normal to ask for help – you do not need to feel ashamed of your symptoms or how you are coping with them, or that you're taking up NHS time when other patients could access the consultation instead.

What to expect from your appointment: the doctor or other clinician (e.g. expert practice nurse) – will want you to give them a good history regarding your periods; so if they are irregular it will be a good idea to bring along a bleeding / menstrual diary – capturing what's happened over the last six months, say. They will want to ask you about your family history relating to any types of cancers or blood clots etc., and the age that your mother was when she experienced her menopause.

They will likely check your blood pressure to review if it's normal, and your weight so that they can work out what your body mass index (BMI) is, to see if you have a normal weight or are overweight or even obese.

These bodily measures will give them more information about why you might be experiencing symptoms of the menopause or how the menopause is impacting on your health and wellbeing.

The doctor or practice nurse might perform an internal examination if you are reporting any irregular bleeding; or organise an abdominal ultrasound scan if that seems to be indicated. They might arrange blood tests too – but remember that the menopause is an informed clinical diagnosis, so taking blood tests is not mandatory. Blood tests that they might consider include FSH (see Chapter 2), iron, vitamin D, B12 and folate, and a full blood count.

Once they have these results, they'll be better able to discuss treatment options with you – maybe changes to your lifestyle habits, prescribed medication like HRT or alternatives to HRT, and what support you should seek at work.

Lifestyle! Lifestyle! Lifestyle!
The **three Ps**: **p**acing, **p**lanning and **p**rioritising should help you to improve your lifestyle habits and think out how you go about organising and re-structuring your days and your week, to accommodate an improved lifestyle.

Pacing is a useful way to manage any activity you have to do. This means breaking an activity down into smaller more manageable chunks and taking a rest in between, rather than just trying to get something done all in one go.

Planning activities ahead of time is really important to understand and control your own limits, rather than letting your symptoms dictate when it's time to stop because you simply can't carry on. Try to do an acceptable amount of physical activity each day and keep this consistent throughout your week, rather than having a few very busy days followed by 'rest' days.

Prioritising is about determining what matters to you, to ensure that you have the energy and control to engage in whatever are the most enjoyable and meaningful activities for you. So that might be: keeping as active as your body allows and doing regular exercise that you enjoy. An achievable regular amount of exercise is better than overdoing it and having to stop for a few days. Go for regular walks – at least 20 minutes per day; or strength training; or take up yoga maybe. Weight bearing exercises should help you to keep your bones strong too.

Food for thought - you might try eating a Mediterranean style diet with lots of plant-based foods that includes a wide variety of vegetables and fruit, wholegrains, nuts and seeds, beans and pulses and fermented foods; and reduce the amount of processed foods, meat, fish, dairy, eggs and sugar in your diet. Avoid caffeine, alcohol and spicy foods too, as they are thought to trigger hot flushes.

Stop smoking if you do and get proper smoking cessation advice from a health professional that will motivate you to quit forever. That should help to reduce your hot flushes too.

Try wearing layered clothing, or use mist bottles or a hand held fan to help to combat any sweats you experience during the day.

Try to keep on top of your stress levels. Notice your triggers and try your best to avoid them. Use a few go-to breathing and relaxation techniques in the moment, and consider adopting some mindfulness and meditation activities into your daily routines – there are some great stress buster apps for these (see Chapter 3 and Chapter 6, for more).

Develop and stick to habits that generate a good sleep pattern: like establishing a cool and dark bedroom, consistent times for going to bed and getting up, limiting your screen use before you go to bed, avoiding caffeine in the late afternoon and evening, take no daytime naps, and spend plenty of time outdoors.

Stay cool at night – sleep in a well ventilated bedroom and wear loose night-time clothes. Take a look at Chapter 3 and Chapter 4 to learn more about what sleep apps you can try too.

Remember that some symptoms associated with the menopause might be caused by other health conditions

So, mood changes like anxiety or depression might not be due to the menopause alone, and may be triggered by other aspects of your life, like your relationships with others or work factors. Similarly, difficulty concentrating or a poor memory might be connected with ageing or life pressures, and not necessarily be linked to the menopause. So, think more widely about any of the symptoms listed in Table 9.1 that you think relate to you, and whether there are other factors in your life that could be accounting for them and take some mitigating actions – don't automatically blame the menopause for all these negative aspects of your life.

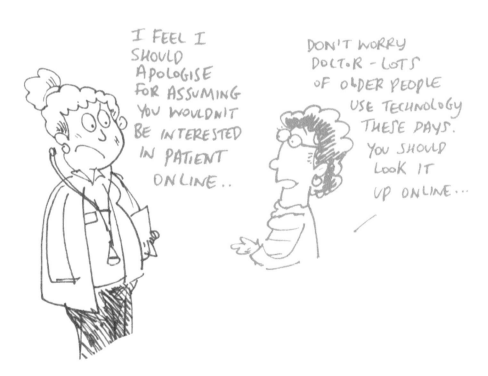

Alternative treatments to HRT going forwards

Selecting an alternative treatment to HRT, or adding it on alongside HRT will depend on your symptoms from the menopause or other health conditions, and your past medical history and experience of previous medication.

Prescribed medication can be very helpful for allied symptoms to the menopause too, like low mood, anxiety or depression (e.g. you might try selective serotonin re-uptake inhibitor drugs such as citalopram, sertraline), hot flushes (e.g. clonidine, gabapentin medication), vaginal atrophy (dry skin) (e.g. moisturisers like oestriol cream or gel) - read more about these options in Chapter 5.

Or you might be offered therapies like Cognitive Behavioural Therapy (CBT), or relaxation – depending on what services are available for a clinician or social prescriber in your general practice to refer you to. A physiotherapist could teach you pelvic floor exercises – so why not ask if your general practice team can refer you?

Hormone Replacement Therapy (HRT): stick with it

Having read Chapter 5 you'll know a lot more about the risks and benefits of taking HRT. You will be prescribed the lowest dose for the shortest possible duration that fits with your symptoms, as you progress. Doctors or prescribing nurses aim to prescribe the lowest dose with maximum efficacy and minimum side effects.

You should expect to have a regular review (initially at three months) to assess the efficacy and tolerability of the treatment(s), adjusting the doses or preparation if needed, and getting advice on stopping HRT if that's justified. Then for ongoing treatment – a review at least six monthly or annually will be the norm, although more frequent reviews may be needed depending on a woman's response to treatment.

Support at work for women experiencing effects of the menopause

So, if you are a line manager or team leader, how can you support your colleagues in your workplace?

- normalise asking for help.
- encourage them to attend a menopausal support group, or try an app.
- link in with local occupational health and wellbeing services and employee assistance programmes.
- extend your team's knowledge about the menopause and create more awareness of how some women struggle with the effects.
- enable access to free training for women to learn how to have safe and effective wellbeing conversations about the menopause and how to access this help.

If you are a line manager consider what reasonable adjustments might support women in the workplace - comfortable work wear/ uniforms, desk fan, flexible working etc. Record menopause-related absences accurately, so your organisation can get a better understanding of the impact menopause is having on colleagues, so that any necessary additional support can be put in place or improved.

How can your organisation or workplace be more menopause friendly?

1. Is there a menopause document / policy in place? If so, are staff aware of it and have they read it?
2. Is there an open and receptive staffing culture around the menopause?
3. Is the right menopause training and support available for staff, whatever their roles or seniority?
4. Is occupational health support available and accessible for staff experiencing menopausal related issues?
5. Is a menopause-friendly uniform / work wear available to staff?
6. Are workplace facilities available that are menopause friendly?

7. Have you considered if temperature adjustments can be made in the workplace and if aids like a desk fan, cold water, and break out space are available and if so, are they accessible?
8. Is there a menopause or wellbeing champion at your workplace as a point of contact?
9. Destigmatise the taboo associated with talking openly about the menopause.
10. Have your organisation's managers (male and female) been advised as to how to make reasonable adjustments that support a positive organisational culture around the menopause?

If the answer is 'no' to any of these ten questions then try to change that ethos in your workplace and start generating the menopause-friendly culture that is needed in your organisation or teams.

If you've problems with your literacy, opt for an Easy Read version

Take a look at the Easy Read leaflets for people with low literacy or learning disabilities. You have to register but it's free and then you can download any of their leaflets. They have one guide on the menopause, amongst others. The website offers you the chance to make donations.

This guide covers:

- What the menopause is

- What happens during the menopause

- What might help you

- Important things to remember (e.g. if you still need to use contraception).

https://www.easyhealth.org.uk/resources/category/118-menopause

Chapter 8

Frequently Asked Questions - and answers from an experienced doctor

Q1: I'm on maximum HRT but still getting hot flushes – have you any advice?

Doctor: Eliminate caffeine AND alcohol in your everyday drinks. Consider discussing changing your HRT medication with your GP or practice nurse, e.g. switch from patches to gel or spray, or vice versa. Ensure oestrogen gel is applied to separate areas and rubbed in fully over a wide area of your skin; or that any gel/spray you've applied is fully dry before you get dressed. If you engage in any energetic exercise/sport then apply the gel /spray after the activity, to allow full absorption.

Q2: My progesterone tablets make me tired/drowsy – what shall I do?

Doctor: Take them just before bedtime and hopefully you won't notice any such side effects from them then during the day.

Q3: I'm getting headaches from my progesterone tablets – what shall I do?

Doctor: Try using the same tablets, in the same dose but placed vaginally. It's probably worth trying the Mirena coil that contains progesterone if your general practice team is able to organise it for you, or fit it in their practice.

Q4: When should my GP refer me for a second opinion from a specialist like a consultant gynaecologist?

Doctor: A GP will usually refer a woman to a gynaecology consultant if she has complex medical problems alongside her menopausal issues;

or fails to respond sufficiently to her HRT treatment; or when side effects persist; or for premature ovarian insufficiency.

Q5: How can I keep my bones strong? I've had my ovaries removed in my 40s and I'm still experiencing all the symptoms from my menopause four years later, especially when I stop my HRT to see if I still need it.

Doctor: Exercise regularly – your joints might be aching more during the menopause – but keep going with the type of physical activities that suit you – it's worth the effort to keep your bones strong and avoid the risk of getting osteoporosis when you're older! If you are a smoker this is your time to QUIT!! And don't forget to check that your usual diet contains sufficient calcium and consider taking a vitamin D 400IU supplement in the winter. The vitamin's protective effect is particularly marked in women of middle-age because declining levels of oestrogen during the menopause can make it harder for the body to produce the vitamin.

Q6: How can I get more help at work for my menopause? When I'm having hot flushes I just must go outside and cool down. My manager asked me really sarcastically the other day if I'd taken up smoking cigarettes. What should I do? Can a GP give me an official note confirming I have got menopausal problems and should be helped to make our workplace more menopausal friendly?

Doctor: Try talking to your line manager first in a one to one meeting, whether they are a man or a woman. You could try an unofficial approach initially, asking for their support for you and other women in your situation – so you can work in a cooler setting, for instance. Maybe pick out a few of your main symptoms as listed in Table 9.1, and discuss how you can be facilitated at work to minimise their effects on you. If that unofficial approach doesn't work, you'll need to seek more official help maybe via your union, or look at the workplace policy and how that is relevant to you and others who are affected by their menopause. Why not talk to others and set up a menopause café that's held once a month to provide support? That might generate shared activities like yoga breathing exercises which should help to reduce participants' menopause symptoms like hot flushes and lower their stress levels.

Even celebrities talk about their menopause these days, and that's helped a lot to get that chat about the symptoms and effects of the menopause and how you can cope, into the media and it's now common to discuss this in public. Good luck!

Q7: I know I'm in the middle of the menopause, but my memory is so bad that my family are asking me if I might be starting with dementia. I'm only 51 years old and my brain fog's been going on and off for a year or so. What do you think – should I get tested for my loss of memory?

Doctor: Having a poor memory or feeling anxious or less able to concentrate, are all common symptoms associated with different stages of the menopause. So, note down your symptoms and how often they happen with some insightful examples from your daily life, and take these notes to a consultation with your GP to discuss what you should do next. Ask if your menopausal treatment can be adjusted, or is there a very unlikely chance that you are developing dementia. Consider trying alternative options like yoga and practise mindfulness to boost your wellbeing.

Q8: The pharmacist said they hadn't got my usual HRT in stock when I went to collect my prescription and when he'd let my GP know, they'd switched my prescription to another treatment – will that have an effect on me?

Doctor: With much more awareness of the effects of the menopause, more women have been seeking treatment and so the demand for HRT has escalated across the UK and pharmaceutical provision of HRT medication has not kept up. Your GP will have opted for alternative HRT medication that's as near as possible in content to the version you usually take. So, give it a try.

Q9: When I first drop off, I sleep deeply but then I wake up half way through the night and find it difficult to get back to sleep again. Difficulty sleeping has only been a problem for me since I started my menopause a few months ago, though it might be my back pain too that's keeping me awake.

Doctor: Well four hours of deep sleep a night is what most humans need. Good sleep hygiene tips include: avoid eating a heavy meal late in the evening, exercise earlier in the day, limit caffeine and alcohol in the few hours before you go to bed. Try and limit noise in your home too so that doesn't wake you up. Make sure you've a cool setting in your bedroom – open your window maybe unless that means you hear a lot of noise from outside. Maybe it's your partner snoring that could be keeping you awake – and you could buy them a gadget to try and minimise their noisy contribution to your night time? Try to avoid watching TV lying in bed or trailing through phone messages and screen shots from your friends. Better to wind down from a busy day by reading a book for a short while, lying in bed.

Q10: What should my diet contain if I want to be as healthy as possible during my menopause?

Doctor: Go for a healthy diet with substantial protein content. Aim for 700-1000mg calcium per day – that might be equivalent to you drinking a pint of milk. All adults in the UK are advised to take a vitamin D supplement over the winter months of 400IU per day (unless of course you have long winter holidays abroad and get plenty of sunshine!). Keep your alcohol down to ideal levels too – maybe stick with a maximum of one drink with alcohol in, each day as a maximum; moving on to some alcohol-free days each week as a regular habit. But don't save up all your alcohol units for the weekend though – spread them over several days instead. You could try cutting caffeine out of your life too – try the decaffeinated options for coffee, tea and fizzy drinks.

Q11: How can I exercise when I am right in the middle of my menopause - getting lots of hot flushes, and sometimes weeing when I'm running?

Doctor: Be kind to yourself, but do as much exercise of whatever types of physical activities that you comfortably can. If your urinary problems persist, see your GP to discuss whether it is the right time for them to refer you to a physio to learn pelvic floor exercises. Yoga exercises should help too. And don't forget that cutting caffeine out or at least reducing the amount you drink should help too.

Q12: Might I be having menopausal symptoms without realising it – as my knee joints are really aching and I'm getting neck and back pains, but I'm still having regular periods at age 49 years old?

Doctor: Yes, your aches and pains might be linked to your menopause- even though you've not realised it's started yet. But there may be other causal factors too, or it might be just normal ageing. Why not go and consult your GP about the musculoskeletal symptoms of your knees or other muscles and joints elsewhere in your body. They might organise some blood tests or maybe a scan or Xray depending on their examination.

Q13: How long should I take HRT for?

Doctor: There are benefits for your heart and bone health up to the age of 60 years old. If a woman is older than 60 years then the risks and benefits need to be carefully (which means clinically) balanced and discussed with the prescribing doctor or nurse. So, your symptom control and enhanced quality of life must exceed the risks – of cancer, or cardiovascular and other health conditions.

Q14: Does HRT cause breast cancer?

Doctor: The risks of getting breast cancer are around 4 extra cases per 1000 women over the course of their HRT treatment. But this is similar to the risk of breast cancer from taking an oral contraceptive. And many adverse lifestyle habits such as smoking and drinking excessive alcohol trigger higher risks of cancer too – so you need to put risks of HRT in proportion and balance the risks and benefits of taking HRT as recommended by your doctor.

Q15: One of my friends who's 47 years old is taking testosterone. Should I be taking this too, as I'm the same age and I've got a low libido.

Doctor: Testosterone is not currently licensed for women. There's no evidence for the use of testosterone except for low sexual desire or loss of libido, associated with distress.

You need to be thinking more widely – have you any problems with your relationship with your partner for instance? Talk through your treatment with the prescribing GP or nurse who'll talk through all the relevant factors in your life – each case is individual, so there's no generic answer.

Q16: I have never had any mental health problems before and suddenly I'm feeling depressed and down, even though nothing much has changed in my work or family lives and I'm happily married. Should I try HRT even though my last period was 12 months ago?

Doctor: Yes, HRT might help – but you won't know until you try it. Other resources like cognitive behavioural therapy (CBT) might help too, or activities like Tai Chi or yoga or other ways of practising mindfulness.

Chapter 9

Make your realistic plan to manage your menopause; ready, steady, nearly go

Start by completing the Table 9.1 below, capturing what symptoms you're experiencing and what actions you'll need to take to overcome them and create a positive plan for a long, healthy life. Complete the boxes below and set out where you are now.

1. Having read the book, what stage of the menopause do you think you are at?

> Write your answer here:

2. What treatment are you taking:

> - prescribed by a doctor or nurse?
>
> - bought over the counter or online?

	Menopausal related symptoms	Tick here
Which of these are you experiencing?	Hot flushes	
	Night sweats	
	Sweating during the day	
	Feeling anxious	
	Poor memory, memory lapses	
	Less able to concentrate	
	Accomplishing less than I used to	
	Feeling depressed or down	
	Mood swings	
	Being impatient with others	
	Wanting to be alone	
	Flatulence (wind) discomfort, bloating	
	Digestive problems	
	Aching in muscles and joint pains	
	Feeling tired or worn out	

Table 9.1. Complete the rows below with as much detail as you like; and fill in the end plan with changes You Will Make!*

	Difficulty sleeping	
	Low backache	
	Headaches (including worse migraines)	
	Reduced physical strength	
	Less stamina	
	Lack of energy	
	Drier skin	
	Increased facial hair	
	Changes in texture or tone of skin	
	Vaginal dryness	
	Involuntary urination when laughing or coughing	
	Frequent urination (weeing)	
	Urinary urgency	
	Avoiding intimacy	
	Decreased sexual desire/lack of libido	
	Change in body odour	
	More brittle nails	
	Breast pain	
	?	

	?	
How will you try to combat your menopausal-related symptoms? Add lots of ideas......		

*This list of menopausal symptoms includes many of those compiled as a 'Menopause-Specific Quality of Life Questionnaire' by Hildith JR and colleagues in 1996, and published by the American Psychological Association; and the range of menopause symptoms relayed on the https://www.menopausenow.com website.

Now move onto Table 9.2 to plan and find doable ways to make possible changes to your lifestyle, home and working lives to minimise the effects that you are getting from the stage of the menopause you're at, and access all the support that is available and accessible to you.

Symbol	Resources you'll need?	What, Where, When? Add lots of details
	Location (where you might walk, jog, run safely, socialise. do Tai Chi)	
	Money/funds (gym, apps worth paying for, exercise equipment at home, sports shoes etc.)	
	Expertise (skills in overcoming barriers, gaining knowledge, enhanced capability and competence e.g. to exercise, do yoga or cook healthy foods)	
	People (adviser e.g. GP, practice nurse, slimming club, dietitian, physiotherapist, psychologist)	
	Reading (tips on the symptoms of the menopause, and treatments or hobbies you could try, what good lifestyle habits are)	
	Information online (access websites, extract tips on beating the menopause, join others on virtual networks)	
	Communication (e.g. newsletter, participate in video-group or menopause café or yoga class to share exercises/ progress on minimising effects of your menopause)	

Table 9.2. Resources you'll need for your action plan to combat the effects of your menopause

	Planning (watch trends in your menopausal symptoms as you change treatments and redress poor lifestyle habits e.g. monitor weight, daily exercise / steps done, sweating, memory)	
	Other actions? E.g. your back up plan….	

So that's it then. You've got all the information you need from this book or the trusted apps and websites and opportunities that we've signposted you to.

YOU CAN DO IT…….go, go, go!!

Appendix   QR Codes for Apps

Balance app

Apple   Google Play   Website

Health and Her app

Apple   Google Play   Website

Caria app

Apple   Website

Perry app

Apple   Google Play   Website

Menolife app

Apple   Google Play   Website

NHS weight loss plan app:

Apple   Google Play

MyFitnessPal app

Apple

Google Play

The NHS Food Scanner app

Apple

Google Play

Couch to 5K app

Apple

Google Play

NHS Active 10 Walking Tracker app:

Apple   Google Play

Drink Free Days app

Apple   Google Play

DrinkCoach app:

Apple   Google Play

These links can also be found at

https://www.raparu.co.uk/menopause

.

Printed in Great Britain
by Amazon

23106280R00066